FINDIN~ ~~~~
LIFE FORCE

Finding peace and embracing life with cancer
Meditations for healing
Real life stories from cancer patients and carers

Caro Jonas
Jane Gillespie

LIFE FORCE CANCER FOUNDATION
Supporting people living with cancer since 1993

Patrons: Gabi Hollows and Professor Michael Friedlander
Compiled by Caro Jonas, Jane Gillespie and Meldi Arkenstall
Edited by Meldi Arkinstall

JoJo
PUBLISHING

Finding Our Life Force
Caro Jonas and Jane Gillespie

Published by JoJo Publishing
First published 2013

'Yarra's Edge'
2203/80 Lorimer Street
Docklands VIC 3008
Australia

Email: jo-media@bigpond.net.au or visit www.jojopublishing.com

JoJo Publishing

Editors: Julie Athanasiou and Meldi Arkinstall
Designer / typesetter: Chameleon Print Design
Printed in China by Reliance Printing.

National Library of Australia Cataloguing-in-Publication entry

Title:	Finding our life force : a practical guide to finding peace and embracing life after a diagnosis of cancer / compiled by Jane Gillespie and Caro Jonas ; edited by Meldi Arkinstall and Julie Athanasiou.
ISBN:	9780987358646 (paperback)
Subjects:	Cancer--Patients--Care.
	Cancer--Patients--Attitudes.
	Cancer--Treatment.
	Quality of life.
Other Authors/Contributors:	
	Jonas, Caro, compiler.
	Gillespie, Jane, compiler.
	Arkinstall, Meldi, editor.
	Athanasiou, Julie, editor.
Dewey Number:	362.196994

www.lifeforce.org.au

Disclaimer

Some of our contributors have written about various methods they used to help them on their cancer journeys. Life Force does not necessarily endorse those methods but we do honour the fact that everyone is an individual and will find their own way of dealing with this very challenging time in their lives. If people express interest in alternative methods of treatment we direct them to the Cancer Council's booklet on Complementary Therapies, copies of which we have on display at meetings. We actively encourage our members to work closely with their clinicians to maximise the benefits of their treatment.

Our goal has always been to provide a safe place for cancer patients, survivors and their carers to work through the emotional impact of living with cancer. Life Force support groups are co-facilitated by trained counsellors and an experienced meditation teacher. All our facilitators have had their own cancer experiences.

Our groups are experiential, where all emotions can be expressed and hopefully normalised. The counselling facilitator undertakes to make sure that everyone is listened to respectfully and no one is told what to do, which lessens anxiety. Each group meeting concludes with a meditation.

Contents

PART 1

Forewords

Michael Friedlander

I have been associated with the Life Force Cancer Foundation since its inception in 1993 and continue to be impressed with the quality of support it provides to patients with cancer and to their families. The people working for Life Force are qualified counsellors, trained group facilitators and an experienced meditation teacher who are totally committed to the cause. They provide individual counselling, weekend retreats in the country and weekly support groups for both cancer patients and their families/carers.

There is very good evidence to support the positive impact of psychosocial services to people with cancer. There are psychosocial guidelines endorsed by the National Health and Medical Research Council (NHMRC) and no one would argue that this is not an important and essential component of cancer care.

Life Force conducts its support groups outside the hospital system and this is preferable to many people and their families. Importantly it is available to all, irrespective of where they have their medical treatment.

Group work can be a very powerful tool in helping people come to terms with the upheaval that a cancer diagnosis creates in many areas of their lives. Attending a support group offers an opportunity to overcome isolation through the sharing of feelings with people who are going through a similar experience. I see the work that the Life Force Cancer Foundation does as an important adjunct to psychosocial support available in hospitals.

The Life Force counsellors work with clinicians and this is consistent with a holistic and collaborative team approach to provide optimal cancer care.

Michael Friedlander PhD FRACP
Director Medical Oncology
Prince of Wales Cancer Centre
Professor of Medicine Conjoint
University of New South Wales

Foreword by Lisa Forrest

I married into the Life Force family. Caro Jonas is my husband's aunt. Jilly Pascoe is his godmother. When I first met my husband almost ten years ago Caro and Jilly asked me if I would emcee Life Force's annual night of Poetry and Prose.

Of course I said yes. It was a pleasure to be asked. And it was the right thing to do. It was the kind of thing where a little effort on my part would go a long way to helping someone else.

Over the next couple of years not only did I hear some of the world's best actors recite their favourite pieces of poetry but also great stories of courage from some of the world's strongest people.

Always mindful of how lucky I was that neither I, nor anyone I loved, had to endure such pain.

Until I wasn't.

In the early months of 2002, my best friend Edwina was diagnosed with a cancer that had started in the breast but by the time the doctors found it was in her nervous system — specifically the fluid of her brain and spine. She was given no time to live. She was 36. With three children aged ten, nine and two.

That year when I hosted the night of Poetry and Prose I truly became one of the Life Force family and no longer one of the lucky ones.

And yet what a privilege it was to be one of the people someone chose to spend time with when they had so little time left.

Eddie and I had many great moments together when she was well. We travelled the world, saw the pyramids, danced to Kylie at Wembley Stadium and shared the joy of our children. But none of those compare to helping her realise her greatest wish when she was fighting the disease.

The cancer moved so fast that very soon after diagnosis she

lost almost complete feeling in her legs. But she refused a wheel-chair, preferring instead to struggle with a walking frame. After seven months of chemo sheer will gave her the remission doctors said would not happen. We seized it. All she wanted was to drive her children to school. For five weeks I drove her to Calvary Hospital in Sydney three times a week so she could have lessons on how to drive as a person with a disability.

The day I took her for the test, I left her at Calvary Hospital and drove away to find a café to wait when I felt a huge kick, right under my ribcage. It was the first real communication I'd had from the unborn child I was carrying. *Hello*, I said. *So you're nervous too, are you?*

Ed got her disabled license that afternoon. Later that night she called me to say that as soon as Lachlan, her eldest, got home from school they went for a drive together from their home in Vaucluse to Watson's Bay. The freedom in her voice will stay with me forever.

We had two years of some of the funniest, challenging and definitely most shocking moments of our friendship. So much of what happened I was prepared for because of my involvement with Life Force.

Eddie passed away in May 2004. She is deeply missed.

For those that are in darkness Life Force provides a light. This book is a testament to the way Jilly, Caro and everyone at Life Force has helped so many of us find a way through the experience of cancer.

PART 2

About the Life Force Foundation

Life Force Philosophy

Meldi Arkinstall

When a human being is unwell the whole human being must be treated, not just the disease. In other words, a holistic approach is needed.

The main beliefs of the Life Force Foundation's philosophy are:

- ‣ Recognition of each individual as a whole human being — physical, emotional, psychological and spiritual.
- ‣ Belief that healing takes place on many levels.
- ‣ Recognition and acknowledgement of the experience of cancer as trauma, and the need for appropriate and supportive care for patients, families and carers.
- ‣ Belief in a balanced approach to health care and the right of the individual to have access to psychosocial support in dealing with illness.
- ‣ Recognition of the value of group work as a powerful tool for healing.
- ‣ In learning how to cope with and transform our feelings of fear, confusion, despair and anger, we have a precious gift — each other.

In 2005 a report submitted to the Department of Health and Ageing, The Cancer Council of Australia put forth the concept that cancer support groups were a powerful way to improve psychological wellbeing. The report, *Building effective cancer support groups,* written by L-M Herron, was the result of a survey of 184 support groups in NSW.

It found that support groups helped people with cancer and their families in the following ways:

- ‣ Reassuring people that their reactions are normal.
- ‣ Providing information about treatment and side effects.
- ‣ Increasing their sense of control.
- ‣ Reducing feelings of isolation through contact with others who understand.
- ‣ Providing a place to express feelings openly, relax, joke and just be themselves.

Countless other academics and authors have espoused the benefits of attending support groups. Although it would be impossible to cite every authority on the subject, of especial note is in an article from the journal *Clinical Oncology* in September 2005.[1] A number of complicated studies were done and databases examined and analysed by researchers at the International University of Catalonia.

They concluded:

> *The results indicate that participation in a support group is associated with significant improvements in a patient's emotional state (depression and anxiety), illness adaptation, quality of life, and marital relationships. Support group participation for patients with cancer has a positive impact in various areas. Nurses should promote participation as a crucial part of their care.*

The Mental Health Weekly reported in January 2004 that support groups were especially useful in promoting the patient's individual resources.[2]

---

1   *Clinical Oncology Week*, (Sept 26, 2005): 100. Cancer Support Groups; Effectiveness of cancer support groups as assessed.
2   *Mental Health Weekly Digest* (Jan 26, 2004):20. Cancer Support Groups; Cancer patient support groups improve quality of life and emotional health.

"Therefore, such groups are helpful not only for the patients, but also for their spouses and other family members. Some research that emphasises the avoidance of feelings, denial of concerns, feelings of helplessness and social isolation are correlated with poorer health outcome and poorer quality of life."

And finally Beverly Zakarian's book, *The Activist Cancer Patient*,[3] agrees with all of the above, "Killing cancer cells is only part of restoring yourself to health. You have to go after what you need in life with the same determination".

She has an interesting perspective on how to manage the impact of cancer on families.

"Discussing your fears with the people closest to you reinforces their own fears, which can only add to yours. Learn, and draw strength and encouragement, from the understanding of others who share what you're going through. Then bring that courage home without the need to unload excess emotion."

---

3 Zakarian, B., *The Activist Cancer Patient: How to Take Charge of Your Treatment*, 1996, John Wiley and Sons 1996.

Meaning behind the Life Force Cancer Foundation logo

In American Indian symbolism, the bear represents courage, strength, protection and unity. This is what Life Force supports people to find within. Caro Jonas, a co-founder of Life Force Foundation, has personal experience of the power of American Indian rituals.

Just as bears hibernate, so should we withdraw from our entanglements and seek refuge within. The answers to our needs and the harmony we seek lie hidden in the silence, within the power of our personal knowing.

Bears also stress the importance of the time to nurture our dreams and aspirations in a quiet period, and to seek ways to own them so they can become practical realities.

The bear is the power of the meditative state — the place of perfect balance and harmony. Life Force group members take time to make meditation a part of their daily routine. Strength comes from looking within.

The female bear is an extremely protective mother to her cubs. She guards them and teaches them intensively for the first six months of their life — a very vulnerable time.

The bear symbolises everything that people need to find when they are feeling vulnerable after receiving diagnosis, undergoing treatment or trying to work out their new reality after treatment ends.

The bear can also be the 'teddy bear', to which we can all relate as a comforter. There are teddy bears present at our group meetings to comfort and help soften sometimes difficult emotional journeys.

The three emblems hanging below the bear, the bottlebrush, wattle and eucalyptus leaves, place the universal bear symbol in an Australian context. They represent the healing powers of the 'bush'; powerful healing flora coming out of the ancient Australian landscape.

Bottlebrush represents serenity and calm, an ability to cope, and helps people move through major life changes. It 'brushes' out the past and allows the person to move on. Wattle gives a sense of optimism and acceptance of the beauty and joy in the present. Eucalypt promotes motivation, direction and life purpose

We have no affiliation with any religion but to be able to access the life force within us, it is fundamental to encourage a belief in something 'more', while respecting each person's interpretation of what that might be. Something more has to have meaning for the individual and could be a specific religious belief or simply choosing to fully live each day to the best of our ability.

How Life Force Began

Caro Jonas

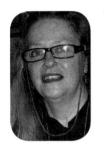

The first Life Force group was set up in Randwick, Sydney in 1993. One of our first group members to attend was a man with prostate cancer. He found the sessions so helpful that he attended every single one.

From there we spread to the inner west of Sydney, and now run groups in Edgecliff and Annandale and off and on in Chatswood. My experience working with all our members has made me believe in the wonder of the human spirit, with all its humour, sadness, determination, resilience, power, energy and truth.

I was diagnosed with breast cancer myself early in 2002. I went through the usual procedures and ended up having a mastectomy and reconstruction at the same time. I had to put into place all the techniques for survival that I had learnt in the previous years. You could say that I was well prepared for the onslaught that was to follow.

Then in 2006, after a routine mammogram, a small tumour was found in my other breast. This time I was advised that a lumpectomy was probably all that was needed. However, the pathology from that was inconclusive and I then opted for another mastectomy. I now live with my prosthesis (called Maud). Not long ago Maud fell from my brassiere into my cats' drinking water as I bent over. One cat, witnessing this strange scene, looked at me with great disdain!

Meditation and visualisation have been an important part of the group process in all the years Life Force has been operating.

15

Professor Leslie Walker, from the University of Hull in England, has said that "relaxation and guided imagery can bring about measurable changes in the body's own immunological defences".[4]

Carl Jung used the human capacity for imagining in a therapeutic way. He distinguished imagination from fantasy, which he saw as 'passive imagination'. He introduced a practice called 'active imagination'. This involved conscious participation in our inner world of images. He encouraged people to 'actively' work with the imagination so as to engage the unconscious with the ego.

Aboriginal healers were concerned with a similar human faculty. They gave it the name 'strong eye'. These indigenous 'shamans' worked to develop greater and greater capacities to bring up images from their subconscious, hold them in their inner gaze, and relate to them. They learned that they had to discriminate between different qualities of images, they had to be careful and selective but they found that they could be a source of inspiration and strength.

Ancient hunters understood the power of this faculty. They saw within themselves, in the realm of imagination, what they wished to happen. They saw, over and over again, the success of the hunt. They ritualised and danced and chanted and 'saw' the desired result before they left. Forming a relationship with positive images they cultivated results, salubrious results, in their 'mind's eye' beforehand and in this way had some control over their destiny. Modern sportsmen and women do the same in the world today; they visualise their desired outcome, which is to win.

When we can go inside and allow images to unfold — for a flower to open in our hearts, to go on a sea voyage, to have a strong warrior protect you, or a healing figure strengthen

---

4   From an article which appeared in *The Sun Herald*, Sydney, Australia on April 16, 2000

you — it is remarkable. Individuals expand by doing this by awakening and reinforcing their imaginative power. They feel that an extra dimension is active within them, and they are buoyed by it. It strengthens them and adds to their being.

In Professor Walker's article he says, "Cancer patients can gear up their immune systems by imagining their bodies waging war on the disease". Referring to a study in which women with breast cancer were asked to visualise white blood cells destroying tumour cells, Walker reported amazing results. Researchers found that the patients had "higher numbers of T-cells, the specialised white blood cells that play a vital role in fighting disease while 'killer' cells, which destroy cancerous cells, become more active".

So, visualising, and visualising 'strongly' (strong eye), can potentially be of great advantage to these patients.

Buddhist monks have cultivated this 'seeing' power for thousands of years. The positive end result of this is re-enforced by Western scientific research into Buddhist meditation.

Research published in *Current Biology* [5] shows that Tibetan monks' meditations help them to 'see the world in a different way'. The scientists found that the monks' skills allowed them to have more control over their mental state and the flow of images passing through their consciousness.

They, with their 'one-point meditation' techniques, were able to maintain their focus on a simple image or thought for much longer than normal; normal people perceive one image, then flip on to another image every couple of seconds. The majority of monks reported seeing just one stable image for five minutes — this is 'strong eye'.

Over the last eighteen years, I have developed many kinds of visualisations designed to expand this same capacity, enabling people to become more empowered.

---

5 From an article in *The Sydney Morning Herald* on Wednesday 8/6/05 by Deborah Smith, Science Editor

One is based on North American Indian culture, others on Aboriginal culture, and yet others on Ancient Egyptian culture. We explore a mansion and sail on a golden galleon. We take trips to islands and to gardens, to taste, to hear, to feel, to cultivate our sense memory, as well as greater creativity. There are many visual journeys that we take — and many more to come.

Rootreat's Main House

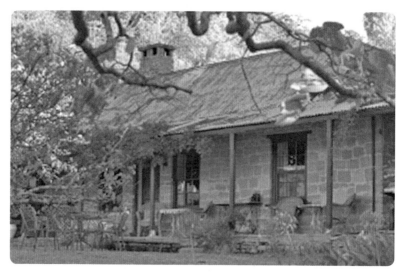

Attending the Life Force retreats at Rootreat B&B allows people to recover their vital energy and has an enormously positive effect on their emotional, spiritual and physical wellbeing.

This has a flow-on effect. It affects their lives and the lives of their families. One of our members said that this power lasted about six months from one retreat to another. A central part of the retreats, which take place over Friday, Saturday and Sunday, is the 'vision quest'.

The power of so-called 'vision quests' started for me about ten years ago when I attended a retreat with a Native American medicine man called Johnny Two-Birds. Jilly and I had booked the weekend together, but her friend Fred Hollows had died and she wanted to go to the funeral in Bourke, so I went off, apprehensively, alone. It turned out to be for the best because I was faced with myself, by myself.

After arriving and some housekeeping, some of us were selected out to go on a vision quest. We were instructed to find a place somewhere outside in nature, a place which felt 'right'. In this place we were to sit and just 'be' and to contact the world immediately around ourselves. It started to rain and I sat in my chosen space (a cave) for many hours feeling uncomfortable and cold.

However, after a while things started to happen. I started to observe tiny things 'happening' around me. I became more conscious of my surroundings and meanings were being conveyed. The cold and uncomfortable wetness disappeared and I was just there in the present moment taking in so much more.

As I sat in the drizzle, I saw an ant struggling along a branch and saw that he was the same as me, coping with the uncertainty of life. Yet, I saw, he had been created and nurtured and even in his smallness had a part to play in the theatre of the universe. The hours sped by and when I heard the drum roll to call us back in, it seemed as if it had been only five minutes.

So much was learnt in my isolation, in my vision quest and this is something we try to achieve on our weekend retreats.

My initial vision quest, and the ones we practise on retreats, although having a power and impact in their own right, are obviously truncated and adapted versions of the traditional North American Indian vision quest.

A vision quest is a rite of passage, similar to an initiation, in some Native American cultures. The quest itself is usually a journey alone into the wilderness seeking personal growth and spiritual guidance from the spirit.

In traditional Lakota culture the Hanblecheyapi, the vision quest, literally means 'crying for a vision', and is one of seven main rites.

It is a period of solitude in which the individual seeks an

inner revelation, a vision, which grants profound meaning and direction to their life. This initiation leads to maturity and an understanding of responsibility to themselves, their society, their natural environment, and their soul. It might take a day, a week, or a month, whatever is necessary to complete the transformation and get the answer one seeks. In Native American traditions, these times of inner trial are marked like passages. Time is set aside to honour them.

Traditionally, the participant finds a place that they feel is special, and sits in a ten-foot circle and brings nothing in from society with the exception of water. A normal vision quest usually lasts two to four days within this circle, during which the participant is forced to look into their very depths.

It is advised that a strong urge to leave the quest area will come to the participant and a feeling of unease may set in. However, the participant normally overcomes this by reminding him or herself of the overall outcome of the quest, causing the mind to stop wandering on random thoughts. Some have claimed grand visions on their first vision quest while others have not. It is an individual experience and often subject to the emotional, spiritual, and physical make-up of the person.

Since early times, humanity has returned to nature to connect with the spirit and to seek answers to problems of the physical realms and their lives. There is something about being alone in the wilderness that brings us closer and more aware of the four elements and our connection to our source. We go to these retreats to seek truths, and perhaps even divine realisation, just as many of the ancient prophets did in their time.

In its own way, the vision quest is an initiation not unlike the days of the ancient mystery school teachings where one learns about one's 'self' and the mysteries of the universe are often revealed to the individual. It is a time of internal transformation and renewal. Who am I? Why am I here? These are the questions that arise.

After our vision quest, some of us were called to participate in a 'sweat lodge'. This entailed sitting in a small tepee with about twenty people whom I had never met before. I was, like the other strangers, dressed only in a towel. We were confined and vulnerable. Water was put onto hot stones to create a hot and close environment.

We weren't able to leave once the entrance was shut and had to decide to go on or to abandon this undertaking. I stayed. Others chose to leave. This confinement lasted for several hours and it wasn't easy.

People talked and cried and shared themselves in a most intense and personal way. I felt extremely claustrophobic and could have panicked, but stayed and gained great strength by breathing, enduring and being in the moment.

On my return drive to Sydney, it started to rain and as I drove in my trusty Kombi van my windscreen wipers failed. It seemed to me this experience was like the 'sweat lodge' all over again. I endured this as well and arrived home ready for a rest and a quiet couple of days. But this discomfort and confrontation with my 'self', although difficult, was full of growth and I was able to take great store from the experience and apply it to my future struggles and to helping others.

There were times ahead, on diagnosis, before results, before operations or simply in the middle of the night, when existence and its sometimes confronting loneliness, was similar to that time in the sweat lodge (when you felt like running, like leaving, although, in reality there was nowhere to go) but stayed and breathed, and found strength in the moment — in the hour of darkness.

One of the most inspirational people to come to the Life Force groups was a woman named Margaret Lindsay. She loved the work we did in the group, the visualizing and the vision quest. She called the groups "her Life Force". She came for six years. She loved the medicine wheel exercises, especially the eagle exercise.

Briefly, this exercise is about being objective in life — about observing yourself impersonally. You look down from a height, like an eagle, and ask, in the midst of an emotion, for example, "What's going on here?" Or "How am I behaving right at this very moment?" The object is to see and act from a clearer, higher vantage point. The visualisation involves rising above a situation, looking down on it and putting things into a wider context. This visualisation, one of my earlier ones, was inspired by Caryn Lea Summers.[6]

She quotes Robert Johnson, in a chapter on objectivity, who says that an individual, "encountering the river of life from the narrow perspective of his own particular river bank may occasionally need to call on his eagle nature to lift his range of vision to take in more of the river, to see all the curves and turns and changes. Then he may put his own situation into better perspective and see other possibilities"[7]. We need, he says, "our eagle natures, especially when we seem caught in a particularly grim bend of the river".[8]

The eagle resonated very strongly with Margaret. When she moved from Sydney to the Central Coast, she chose her new house because it had an eagle as a door knocker. She took it as an omen.

When Margaret was going through the dying process she held on and wouldn't let go. It wasn't until her husband, Jack, who was sitting by her side, urged her to let her eagle 'take her', did she let go and she passed away. Her eagle, which she found in her imagination and which resonated very personally with her, helped her just when she needed it. It carried her off. It

---

6 *Circle of Health — Recovery Through the Medicine* Wheel p30-32, The Crossing Press, Freedom, CA, 1991
7 Ibid p30
8 Ibid

helped her in her time of need. Because her imagination had been awakened, expanded and strengthened over time, it was her saving grace in her most profound time of need, on her death bed.

It must be said that Margaret's use of the eagle was, ultimately, different from the original intent of the exercise. She took the image and used the power and resonance of the eagle for her own purposes. It 'carried her away', as it were, long before it did at her death.

This, of course, is perfectly acceptable. People's imaginary facility is their 'own', and the joy for them is to see that this 'new' and 'developed' capacity is there to add to their being — to enrich them and support them.

PART 3

Meditations

Benefits of Meditation

Put simply, meditation is the method of bringing a scattered and disorganised mind into a state of peace, quiet and tranquillity.

The word meditation is derived from two Latin words, 'meditari', meaning to think, to dwell upon, to exercise the mind, and 'medha' which means to heal. Medha is derived from the Sanskrit word meaning 'wisdom'.

This word origin gives an insight into the intention of the practise of meditation. It is built around an inner focusing.

This inner looking supports a moving away from the distractions of the outer world with its noise and multiplicity towards a more subtle and neglected part of ourselves. Inclusion, and cultivation, of this 'forgotten' part completes us, makes us more whole.

This other place can also be discovered as a place which possesses a mysterious wisdom. This relationship, of our conscious part with our unconscious part, can be a salubrious one, bringing a calmness of mind and more 'solid' feelings.

When gained these solid feelings within us act as a deep support, and can lead us to wholeness or health.

In meditation we train ourselves to become more and more aware. We aim to become more conscious. Observing your breath, or listening to birds more closely, or becoming more aware of the subtleties of light or colour, for example, are all examples of what we can do to move towards having greater consciousness.

In time, as we cultivate the above, we become better at sensing and receiving the subtle gentle energies that are active within us. We can then see that this gentle and subtle presence within us is an astounding part of us that has been hitherto neglected.

There are many ways to achieve the desired ends of meditation. Some meditation involves a 'mantra'. This is a specially given word which directs the mind inwards. Intoning this sound within acts as a focus for the mind, and often has a special quality of sound or vibration which itself has a healing aspect.

One keeps returning to the intoned sound and returns again and again as we orientate ourselves in a new direction.

We can through this, 'centre' ourselves and move towards a potential process of healing.

In a much more simple way, as opposed to repeating an intoned sound, we can gain much by just being more deeply aware, and in touch, with the breath and the rhythm of the breath.

By calming the mind and body, we learn not to be disturbed by the images which exist in our subconscious and which are available to us; we find another part of us which is 'our' place, which is as much a part of us as our body or our conscious outer mind.

Scientifically speaking, Dr Ramesh Manocha[9], in studies at the University of NSW, showed that meditation is good for the health.

He found that 'finding a mental silence' has been proven to reduce stress and anxiety, and to improve and increase our ability to adopt and adapt. There is evidence he said, "That it can improve blood pressure and the physiological effect of stress by decreasing the level of stress hormone in the bloodstream".

Furthermore, he says, that it may also, "Improve the strength of the immune system and reduce the physical aspects of disease". He surmises that, "It probably works by acting on the emotional centres in the brain".

Visualisation is another form of meditation. This method is the one I use in the Life Force groups.

---

9   Interview — 7.30 Report ABC TV 2002, Location http://www.abc.net.au/7.30/content/2002/s499180.htm. Broadcast 07/03/2002

Our ability to visualise is so commonplace to us that we are rarely aware of it or how fundamental it is to our lives.

It is a magnificent gift.

When we simply go on a trip to the shops or plan a trip we 'see' where we're going or what we'll buy long before we leave to complete our 'thought-out' action.

We use this 'visualising' in most of our actions. When we don't this is when we find ourselves 'blindly' doing things.

When we become more conscious of this mental/emotional planning process within us we may begin to see that it is a sacred, even miraculous function that we have. This can change us in a most positive way.

We may, furthermore, come to see that we can cultivate this marvel and increase our capacity to use the facility. When we do this we begin to potentially increase our quality of life, our wellbeing and our health.

Carl Jung's therapeutic use of the imagination is well known.

He distinguished imagination from fantasy which he saw as ordinary, passive imagination. He introduced a practice called 'active imagination'.

This involved conscious participation in our inner world of images. He encouraged people to 'actively' work with the imagination so as to engage the unconscious with the ego.

For us it can be wonderful, expansive and exciting to begin to develop a more heightened ability to visualise.

It can be a most beautiful thing to see and cultivate within us a quiet place, such as a healing stream where we can lay and be cleansed and calmed.

It can be reassuring to see and engage with a wise and loving sage — a sage who simply personifies our own inner 'wisdom'. We can engage with an endless number of images, things and people. The possibilities are endless. All these things are part of us; we can either assimilate them or not. We choose. We undertake when we do this, a potentially remarkable experience.

Great things can be achieved as we develop a 'strong eye'. We can attain personal growth. We can discover something exciting and deeply personal, an idiosyncratic creativity and our individuality. Most importantly, as modern medicine and science sees the power of this inner focusing, we can discover for ourselves our own inner wisdom and power.

This gives the individual who may be sick, and who is by necessity, always in others hands, a sense of control and their own 'power'. They can direct their own thoughts and develop inner strength.

This power to act and be active in their struggle to be whole again is incredibly empowering.

Preparing for Meditation

The use of the meditations in the book is a very free and relaxed undertaking. Individuals should choose how they want to approach this activity according to their different needs, situation, personalities, habits and preferences.

General advice will follow but it is important that you approach this with deep calm and no anxiety.

Setting Up

To set up for meditation:

- Choose a favourite time either day or night and keep it regular. Create a routine.
- Find a favourite spot one that you can go back to each time and feel as though it is your place, preferably a room that you can close off.
- Dim the light. A little candle to focus can be helpful.
- Make sure that watches and phones and technology are left behind.
- Wrap yourself in a blanket or cover your lap with a beautiful cloth.
- Burn some incense or rub a fragrant oil on yourself.
- You can turn on some soft music but it must be non intrusive.
- Either sit on a nice comfortable and favourite chair or lie down on a cloth of your choice.

Approach to the Meditations as a Series

Different approaches suggested:

Take each series, once a day, over a ten week period. However, if you want to move on to the next meditation after four or five days, do so — the rules are for you to decide. Don't create anxiety with too much rigidity — find a 'way' for yourself.

Always start in a comfortable position with your eyes shut and then concentrate for 5 minutes on your breathing. Focus on the in breath then focus on the release of the breath. This will induce a sense of relaxation and also enhance visuals. Take your time and enjoy it. You may come up against your impatience — work gently against it with your deep and slow breathing.

Over a period of time the ability to visualise will grow. So, be patient and non-judgemental. Persist with kindness and a deep trust in yourself — and you will develop your relationship with the process different and unique to you.

After breathing for five minutes bring your focus down into your heart and lungs and use the breath to keep your focus in this vital area as this is where you will create your visualisation.

Some people visualise better than others — some 'see' things clearly while others are slower in getting to clear images. It doesn't matter, work at it and you'll find your own way.

When you start each new meditation you will of course have to have the book on your lap. You can look down to read the action happening and then close your eyes and see it within you. Then look down and read the next part of the journey. Take your time; there is no rush.

Finish the journey this way each day until you can anticipate more of what's coming. Eventually you will easily glide through but if you have to go back to the book it is okay.

Let other images come into your journey (or smells or sounds). Let them embellish your journey. Stay with things or change events. This can be a moving world of wonder.

Twenty minutes a day is enough each time but you can extend this time if you are feeling solid.

Once you repeat this exercise and cultivate a 'strong eye' (an ability to see more strongly within you) then try to take the 'taste' of the found tranquillity into events in your normal life. At first this may be mundane things like shopping or talking to a friend. Eventually, though, this 'taste' can be taken into more stressful situations.

It is important to note that not all people experience this 'visual' in the same way. You will have your individual way of experiencing it.

Some people 'see' their images, others may not see the images, but they smell, taste, or feel things — and this is okay. Just visualise and enjoy the journey in your own way. Whatever way, your ability to experience will get better the more often you do the exercises.

Cultivate this place of healing; this place of the 'strong eye'.

Each of these meditation series will be heightened if you accompany your visual journey with some concrete 'homework'. Start a creative project such as a collage — so that each week you add an image or many images to match your visual journey. It could be in any form — a mandala or square or oblong. It could be on paper or cloth or whatever you choose. It is your personal project and can be laid out (or not) near your 'ritualised' space.

You may be visited by images which rise up from your subconscious. You can use these images to create your own drawing collage or you may like to download images from the internet or cut them out of magazines. It doesn't matter. It is your project. By doing this you will establish a wonderful relationship with an inner and forgotten, yet deeply important part of you.

This creative action, inspired by your own personal meditations, shouldn't be underestimated in your healing journey. Try it and see for yourself.

At the end of each meditation series there should be a deeply personal and wonderful work of art — your very own work.

Golden Galleon Meditation Series

Week 1: *Inheriting the Ship*

Week 2: *The Island of Trees and Forest*

Week 3: *The Island of Soft Waters*

Week 4: *The Island of Swirling Winds*

Week 5: *The Island of Meadows*

Week 6: *The Island of Pure Sounds*

Week 7: *The Island of Gentle Sands*

Week 8: *The Island of Oneness and Enlightenment*

Week 1

Inheriting the Ship

Preparation for the Journey

You are on a beach. A longboat moves slowly towards the shore. Six men are rowing. They wear the leggings of the time. They are all good men and women. They give you the deeds to the boat.

You look and see a huge Spanish Galleon.

They take you to reclaim your ship. You feel secure. It seems right. There is nostalgia, as though it is something that is rightfully yours. You are amazed and excited.

You don't worry that you are to leave on the ship. You know that you will be safe and that you will not be missed and will return at the right time. All is well.

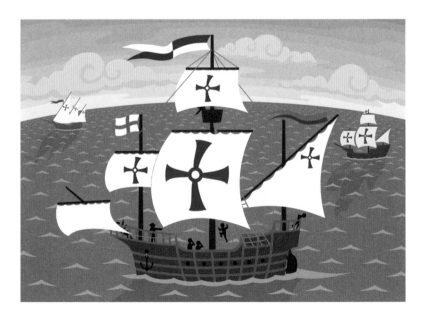

You row back to the ship, board and are introduced to the massive crew. They cheer you. You are the captain and they are there to serve and protect you.

The ship hasn't sailed for a while. All are working hard to repair, renew, and service the ropes, the planks and the sails. There is now much hard work to do. You join in and take much pleasure from this preparation.

Working with your team of men and women you work on the following things:

- Food and supplies are taken on board.
- The galley is stacked with boxes of food.
- Sails are checked.
- Decks are painted and waterproofed.
- Sails are mended and checked.
- Anchors are checked.
- Rudder and steering are checked.
- Sleeping compartments are checked.
- Medicine chests are filled.
- Navigation instruments are checked.
- The mast is checked and secured.
- The decks are scrubbed.

You are preparing for a beautiful journey. You work hard. You feel no fear but you feel great confidence and excitement. All the people on the ship support you and you feel very safe.

Week 2

The Island of Trees and Forest

The Feet: Connecting with Stable Reality

You are taken to an island. You are taken ashore by longboat. As you glide you begin to focus on your breathing.

Take your time as you head towards the shore to connect with your breathing. You are being rowed slowly but steadily. You breath matches the dipping of the oars in the water. It is slow and rhythmical, and your breathing is in tune with it.

You begin to feel relaxed and at ease. You land on the shore and begin to walk up the beach. You see many tall and beautiful trees. You walk towards the trees. As you walk to the centre of the island you begin to see that there is a forest of very tall and strong trees. You walk amongst them and you marvel at their

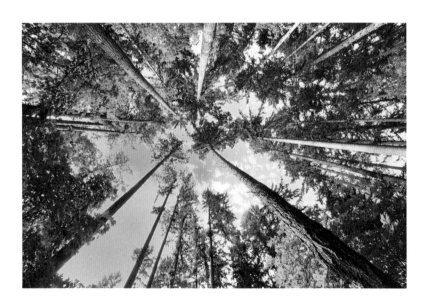

height. You marvel at the strength of their roots and of their ability to hold these mammoth trees strongly in the ground.

You spend some time touching the trees. You feel the many types of surfaces. You touch the leaves, smell the many smells, listen to the sounds of the wind through the trees and hear the birds sing. You look at the many insects, the nests of the birds, the spider webs, the insect holes, the ants on the trees and on the ground. Touch the moss. Sniff it. Feel its moisture. Rest on the moist ground and experience being deeply in that moment.

As you do this, you take off your shoes and rest your feet on the soil between the roots.

You begin to feel from your whole being, and then through your feet, a great connection to the earth. You feel your energy go deep beneath the ground, as deep as the roots of the trees.

It gives you great strength. You gain great stability from this. You feel deeply connected to this earth, to this reality, to this world. Strong winds wouldn't shift you. You would sway but you would never fall. Feel that strong resilience deep inside you.

Close your eyes and enjoy this feeling of strength, of connectedness, of stability within this *real* world. When you open your eyes you find that you have been lifted up into the highest tree, on a solid platform. Safe you sit comfortably and are stunned by the silence. You sit and enjoy the beauty and the stability of this silence.

You are then taken down and return to the beach, then to the boat and back to your ship.

Week 3

The Island of Soft Waters

The Pelvic Area: Creative Inspiration

You are taken to another island. As you glide in the longboat you get in touch with your breathing. By the time you get to the shore you feel deeply relaxed. Take your time. Rowing to the shore and breathing with the slow dipping of the oars should take some time.

As you walk up the beach you see that it is a rocky place but with rocks that are smooth and easy to walk on. These rocks dominate the landscape. Running through the area of smooth rocks is a gently flowing watercourse. It runs in a gentle stream but flows over a large area of the rocks so that it creates endless rock pools. You look into one or two and see lichens and small

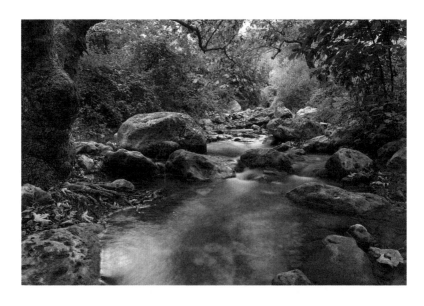

creatures swimming. You see life. You begin to see that they are like mini-worlds.

You spend your time looking, sensing the smoothness of the rocks and the warmth of the sun within them. You realise that the sun is actually within the rocks and therefore in all things around you. You look at them all; the water, the plants, the birds and small animals.

You see that this is a big version of the rock pool. All connected to the sun, even the shade. You begin to feel connected to all that is around you. And begin to feel a deep love for the world, for this creation. You sit and enjoy. It fills you with a wonder. You stay for a long time with this.

You then walk back to the shore, to the longboat and crew and return to your ship. On your journey back, you feel a creative urge deep within, which you take with you to create something. You are filled with great creative energy.

Week 4

The Island of Swirling Winds

The Navel and the Solar Plexus: The Will to Do

You are taken to another island. As you are taken to the island in the longboat, the rhythm of the dipping oars relaxes you and you become attuned to your breathing. By the time you arrive at the shore you are deeply relaxed. Take time to travel with the dipping oars.

As you alight from the boat you look up and see a great mountain in the centre of the island.

You know that you have to climb this mountain and that you have a great challenge ahead. With courage you relax and decide to enjoy this climb and are determined to learn all that you can from it.

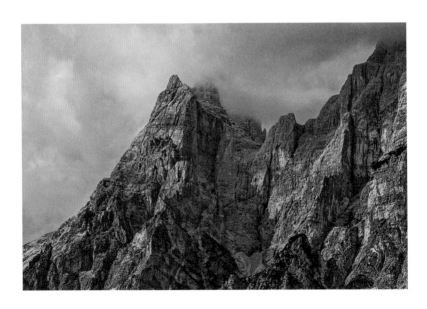

As you climb you begin to feel a growing excitement. You see that as you climb you are going deep within yourself and finding something that you've lost. You don't know yet what it is but you know that it is something important and your heart warms to the task of getting to the top.

When you arrive at the top you rest and breathe. As you sit there looking up to the sky you see a storm build in the huge sky above you. You are safe and are simply observing this wonderful display.

You see great lightning filling the sky and a great area of swirling wind. It is powerful but not frightening. The wind and the lightning join one another and there is great energy and power.

As you watch you see what has been lost. It is a talent that you had forgotten. Something you felt long ago that you could do or dreamt of doing. Maybe something that you dreamed of doing but didn't because you got lost in a sea of criticism, by others or by your own inhibiting voices or maybe the realities of life stalled these aspirations and they were forgotten. Until now when they come flooding back to you. You, with joy and safety, realise that it is possible to take the energy of the storm, the winds, the lightning into yourself, into your navel and then your solar plexus. This energy can be used to will what you seemed to have lost.

You feel that you've touched the very core of your being. These deep and complex feelings that you journeyed towards seemed overwhelming at first, but now you realise they are okay.

You see that you can not only weather these storms but use them, draw energies from them, to achieve forgotten dreams. You walk down the mountain to put things right and to do one thing that you've always wanted to do or even several things.

You return to the boat and are taken to your ship. You are now, deep within yourself, steeled for action. And something lost is restored.

Week 5

The Island of Meadows

The Heart: The Loving Connection

You are taken to another island. As you are taken in the longboat, the slow rhythm of the dipping oars gets you in touch with your breathing. You relax deeply.

When you land, you walk up the shore and in the middle of the island you come to a beautiful gentle meadow.

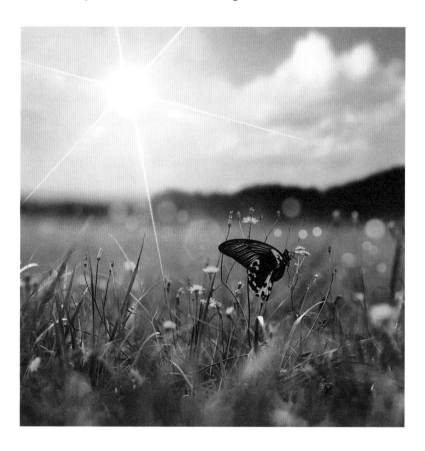

You roam in this meadow enjoying its many wonders; the soft grass, the babbling stream, the light through the trees, the tiny lizards and the sound of the wind in the trees. You explore many things, the sights, the things to touch and the smells.

You experience:

- Hearing a humming bird at a flower. You hear its wings vibrate and flutter.
- Seeing the different colours of the flowers with their variations of size and structure.
- Smelling gardenias, pine needles and cones, lemon-scented grass, salt air and the coolness of the running water.
- Tasting fruits or berries on the trees.
- Drinking milk from a coconut.
- Seeing the dappled light on the trees and the ground.
- Hearing different sounds of animal, birds and rustling of leaves.

You spend time experiencing even more.

As you experience all this, you feel that time slips away and there is just this moment. You experience 'patience' where there is nothing but this moment and these experiences. You truly experience all these wonders around you. Your heart grows warm and this warmth is deeply satisfying.

A tiny flame starts in the heart area. It burns within you as you go back to the shore, back into the small boat and then finally back to the ship.

Week 6

The Island of Pure Sounds

The Throat: Uttering the Truth

You are taken to another island. As you are taken in the boat towards the shore you notice that this time it is very cold. The climate has changed. The conditions are arctic. You are warm and cosy. Your breathing aligns with the oars dipping in the water. You are deeply relaxed when you step onto the icy shore.

You walk up the embankment onto an icy landscape. It is white, beautiful and empty. There is silence as you cross this amphitheatre of white. You have spikes underneath your shoes and so are surefooted. There is no danger.

You stand in this pure landscape and look in wonder. It is empty. It is shining with the sun. You stand and enjoy the

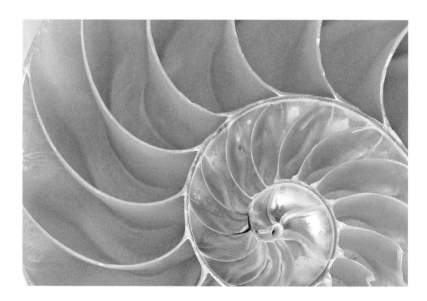

silence until there is an urge to utter a sound. It is a sound that starts in your throat. It starts as a red colour and comes out through your mouth as a sound. It is your unique cry. It is your sound that expresses the pure truth of your whole life, of this moment, of you. It is the sound of your pure essence.

After you express this sound it emerges into the pure air of the natural icy theatre as a blue colour. This colour whirls around the huge space. There is cleanness, clarity, purity and there is a silence which you take some time to enjoy. Stay with the silence for a long time.

You then return to the boat and return in silence to your ship.

Week 7

The Island of Gentle Sands

The Third Eye: Surrender and Bliss

You are taken to another island. Your breathing blends with the dipping oars. When you arrive on the shore you are deeply relaxed.

As you walk up the beach you see that it is a desert island. It is pre-dawn. You can see but only just. There is only sand. You walk into the centre of the landmass and experience the desert sand.

The environment, although sparse, is a gentle one, the temperature is pleasant and the sand easy to walk on. You walk to the centre of this huge sand mass. It is a gentle environment. You see a big white circle drawn in the sand. You sit in the middle of the circle.

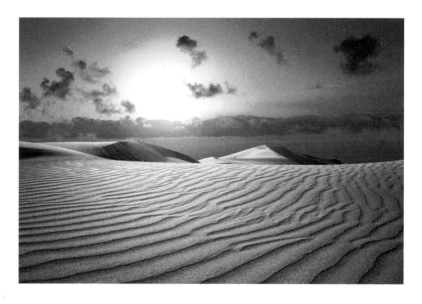

You feel comfortable as you experience this emptiness.

You face the sun which is now beginning to rise over the horizon. As the first light appears it streams over the land and gently touches you. You feel the warmth. The light streams over your body and begins to flow gently and lovingly into your third eye between your eyebrows in your forehead.

This third eye is filled with light. This part becomes filled with gold and passes through all the cells of your body. A beautiful golden light gathers and you feel bliss pass through your body.

The sun, through its light and heat, energises you and you become part of it. You and the sun's rays are one. You stay with this feeling for a few moments before you return to the boat and then finally to your ship.

Week 8

The Island of Oneness and Enlightenment

Merging with the Infinite

You are now sitting in a comfortable chair. The air is clear. The temperature is mild.

You find yourself on the original beach looking out to sea. Small waves are slapping softly on the shore.

You close your eyes and put your mind into your feet. When you do this you become aware that the ship, *The Golden Galleon*, is now tiny and located within your body. Your mind is directing the ship.

The ship begins to journey within you and to all the islands that you have just travelled. It starts in your the feet at The Island of Forest and Trees and as the ship passes through your

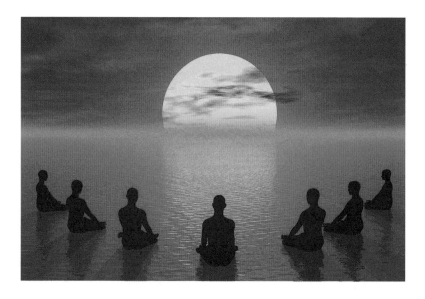

feet, you recall your deep incision into the ground when you stood by the trees. You recall the joy of this connection with the concrete world. You recall the feeling of security you had.

The ship now travels to the pelvic area. You recall the Island of Soft Waters with its smooth rocks, rock pools, island animals and the birds. You recall your connection with the world around you and you recall the feeling of the love in your heart and your creative inspiration.

The ship then moves up to the naval area. You see the Island of Swirling Winds. You recall the storm, the winds and the lightning. The ship moves deeper into your solar plexus. You recall the forgotten talents and neglected dreams you recovered, the gathering of energies, and your efforts to restore these precious things.

The ship now moves to your heart and you see the Island of Meadows. You see the gentle landscape. You are again in a timeless moment and your heart fills with love as you experience all the beauty around you.

Now the ship moves up to your throat and you find yourself in the Island of Pure Sounds. You see yourself in the icy, blue and sparse arctic. You hear your unique cry and then a silence. You feel satisfied and in touch with who you are.

The ship now moves up into your third eye. You recall the warmth of the sun touching you as you sit in the desert landscape. You recall the light entering your forehead and filling you with golden light. You recall how you felt — as though you and the sun were one.

The ship now, finally, moves to the crown of your head. You see another island, a beautiful island that feels like home. It feels right to be there. It is the 'Island of Connection'. You find yourself back in your chair and a great warmth and light fills your body. The crown of your head glows. You move back down through your body and you glow with warmth. All the islands, all these different centres shimmer with their different experiences. You feel whole.

The Meadow Series of Meditations

Week 1: *Starting the journey*

Week 2: *Fear to Peace: The Dove Takes Your Fear*

Week 3: *Pain to Comfort: Climbing the Mountain*

Week 4: *Depression to Happiness: Storm Clouds Lifting*

Week 5: *Anger to Serenity: Smashing the Rock*

Week 6: *Self-doubt to Confidence: The Little Self and the Big Self*

Week 7: *Hate to Love: The String and the Heart*

Week 8: *Weakness to Strength: The Mouse and the Bear*

Week 9: *Terror to Calm: The Storm on the Lake*

Week 10: *The Wonderful Conclusion*

Week 1

Inheriting the Meadow

The Start of the Journey

Every good deed that you have done has been noted and recorded. As you inwardly acknowledge this, a piece of land is given to you as a gift for all your past good works. You have been rewarded. You must now explore, improve and expand this new land.

This is a very large piece of land, about the size of a football field. It is surrounded by a large, unkempt hedge. The entrance to the area is through an old iron gate. It is old and creaky, and needs repair. It is rusty, it squeaks, and doesn't close properly. It has been neglected as have many things within the rectangle of land.

The ground itself is hard and undernourished. After years of neglect it is full of rubbish. It has been used for years as a

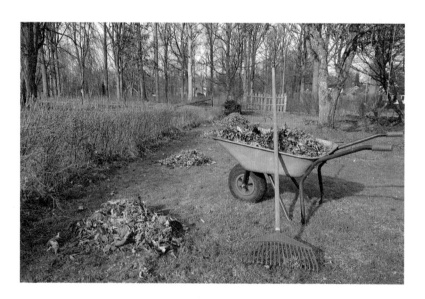

dumping ground. It is littered with old cars, tyres, scaffolding, bikes, clothes and white goods.

The object of this exercise is to transform this desolate and neglected place into a clean and ordered paradise. It must be turned, in our imaginations, into a place where you can come at any time to find shelter, peace, tranquillity, safety, inspiration and healing.

In this space, in this inner world, our disordered state must be seen, acknowledged, and then re-ordered and transformed. From this neglected land you are to create a sacred space.

Cleaning the Space

Get to work. Gather your tools. Remove the rubbish. Sweep. Fix and oil the gate. Fix the lock.

You find a key and it is the only one that opens and locks the gate. It offers security. Put it in a safe place on your being.

Mulch and compost is made. You work hard. You sow seeds. You build a garden. It is a garden of your own choice. The type of garden comes from a deep inner quality that is your true self. You give expression to yourself as you design and build this garden.

It can be an herb garden, a wild cottage garden, a Persian garden or an Australian native garden. You choose from deep within your nature.

You seed the new garden beds and water them. Things can grow at any speed you choose. They can come straight up as you plant them. All this is up to the power of your imagination. It is a deep and given power. You create your own world — your own inner garden of the mind.

Hedges that surround the land are shaped after years of running wild. They are now contained and shaped. The hedges give total privacy. It is a private, secure and sacred space.

Enjoying the fruits of your labour

Now after all the cleaning, planting, watering and shaping you stand and look at your handiwork.

There is a wonderfully satisfying scene in front of you now. There is now a meadow in front of you full of colour, life and energy. There is power in the scene. You feel enjoyment and inspiration. Everything sparkles in the sunlight. Wonderful scents linger in the air. The sounds of bees buzzing and birds singing meet your ears. Butterflies flutter while they display their vivid colours. Tiny animals look at you with curiosity and with affection. The gate is newly painted and no longer squeaks.

You now walk in your meadow. You smell the flowers and the mulch. You touch, feel and roll on the ground. You look at the light as it falls and creates mottled light. You see and differentiate the different colours.

You go to the middle of the meadow and lie on the soft grass. You drift off in total security and fall into deep rest.

There is no one to disturb you. All negatives leave you and go into the compost heap where they undergo transformation into useful fertiliser which will feed your red roses. You think of these flowers in the centre of your garden and experience deep love.

Maintain this love in your heart. See the red colour of the rose. Do this for several minutes. Leave by the gate when you arise. Lock the gate behind you. As you leave a gentle rain falls on your meadow.

When you return next week it will be full of growth and wonder. It awaits you always anytime, night, day or during times of trial. This garden is a gift to you.

Week 2

Fear to Peace: The Dove Takes Your Fear

You now return to the meadow that you inherited and prepared last week for occupying. You arrive and look through the gate. You see the garden's shapes and colours.

You are about to enter and you realise what you are wearing. It is a black cloak. You perceive that it represents a fear state that you carry with you. You accept this state and want to explore. The cloak is made out of beautiful and very light fabric. It is so light that it floats as you walk.

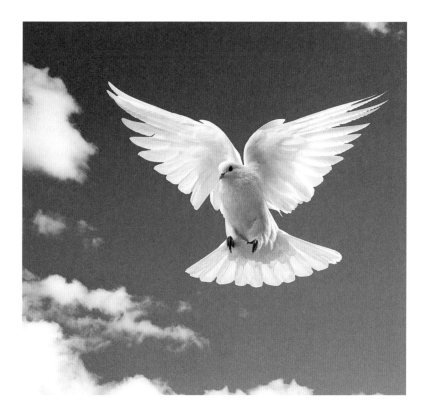

The cloak has a hood which covers your head. You look down to the ground as you walk. You walk with fear. You are afraid as you enter your meadow.

The gate opens easily. Your meadow lies in front of you even more beautiful than when you were last here. It rained as you left and the growth is very impressive. It is lusher and full of colour. However because of your state you don't see its richness and its energy.

You don't see the life in front of you. You are paralysed. You think nothing and desire to do nothing. You sit in a corner of the meadow. You are sad, lonely and depressed. All seems lost.

You stay in this state. You look at yourself and realise that you are watching yourself from a high vantage point. You see that the state is within you but that you are able to look down on it and watch it run its course. You watch it as it runs and runs and then begins to lose energy.

As you do this a beautiful dove appears. It brings a message to you. It says, "All is not lost. Look around you, at the beauty and the endless change of things. There's not a moment to waste. The darkness will lead you nowhere. Look towards the light".

The dove flies around and around you as a beautiful joy comes to your heart. The wonderful creature then drops a white gossamer wrap onto you. You are covered with the softness of the white cloth. The dove coos and you hear this cooing deep within your soul.

The dark, immobilising energy, along with the hooded cape have now gone. The white wrap is now around your shoulders and from it passes creative and shining energy which fills your heart with joy. You visualise future plans, a light passes into your mind and you see clear pictures, scenes playing out of future possibilities.

Being in this moment dissolves time. Time is no longer important. You simply are.

You enter eternity.

You take the joy in your heart, the clear inspiring images in your head and explore the meadow again. Now you have a spring in your step. You smell flowers, listen to the birds' song, hear the sound of the little stream running and smell the grass.

You then lie down in the soft grass and sleep deliciously. When you wake you leave through the gate taking with you the beautiful shawl which is now yours to give you a strong loving heart and a mind full of wonderful images, any time you feel the pull of darkness.

Week 3

Pain to Comfort: Climbing the Mountain

Now that you have tasted the meadow you realise that you are unable to get to it. You can't seem to find your peaceful place. You seem paralysed. What is stopping you is that you are in great pain — physical, mental and emotional. You can hardly walk so great is your pain. Thinking and feeling are difficult for you. Moving seems impossible.

As you stall and are immobilised the dove from the last exercise flies over and drops a small purple basket into your lap.

In the basket is another message. It tells you to look at the horizon. As you do this you see a large mountain. You are told that this is the mountain of pain.

The message says that if you can climb to the top of this great mountain there you will find your meadow again. It says however that you need to travel and endure a little to get there.

You decide to go because you trust the message from your experience with the white cloth. You also have tasted the peace and security of your meadow and are now willing to make this effort to get there.

You feel rightness about this journey. As you look up towards the snow covered peak of the mountain you are no longer paralysed by fear but feel a steely determination. You are buoyed by the challenge of climbing out of yourself. You are taking the initiative. Your fate is now in your hands.

You walk along a road that leads to your mountain. You walk and walk until you come to the foot of the mountain. At the base of the mountain you find three baskets.

The first basket is marked 'bodily pain'. The second is marked 'mental pain' and the last is marked 'pain of the heart'.

You place the small baskets over your shoulder and begin to climb.

You climb and climb. The incline increases and your body begins to ache. Your lungs ache, your legs and back start to ache, your head aches as do your eyes. Your whole body starts to ache. You are in physical pain. You stop and begin to place each pain, mentally, into the basket marked 'bodily pain'.

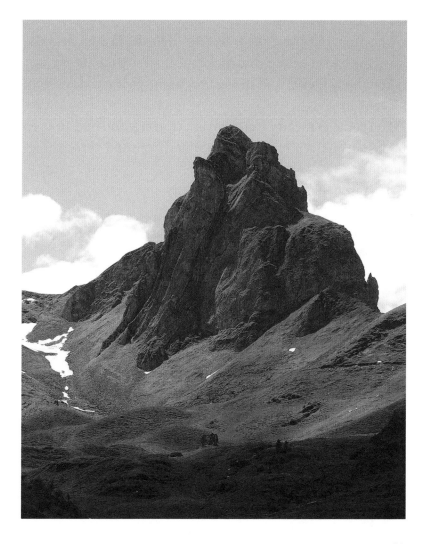

You then leave the basket behind.

As you climb the incline increases and you have to work harder. You begin to have doubts about the undertaking. You have negative thoughts; you are flooded with painful thoughts, horrible future possibilities and memories. You stop and mentally place these mental pains, one by one, into the basket marked for them.

You then leave the basket behind.

As you climb it becomes really steep.

As things get harder your heart fills with dread, fear and other negative feelings.

You stop and place these feelings into the last basket. You leave the basket behind and make the final steps to the top.

Your body is clear and strong now, as are your mind and your heart.

You come to the top and there is a clearing. You find an open basket in the centre of the space and you find three things inside it:

> ‣ A soft blanket of many colours that you fold around yourself to heal your body.
> ‣ A beautiful poem which brings harmony and delight to your thoughts.
> ‣ A tea set and baby cakes which bring great solace and induce lovely feelings.

As you partake of these three things you close your eyes and you find yourself suddenly back in your meadow. It has never been far away.

You are now free of pain. Your body is whole and well, your mind is full of beautiful and positive thoughts and your heart is solid and full of love. You light a flame and a candle is lit in your heart. This flame burns deeply and warmly no matter what happens to you.

Pain has become, through your efforts, comfort.

You lie down with your blanket and fall into a delicious sleep — safe in your meadow once again. The struggle to get there has made this special place even more special.

You wake and go out the gate knowing that even when the meadow is hard to find you can always go back there. You also know that the blanket, poetry, tea and baby cakes are there for you.

Week 4

Depression to Happiness: Storm Clouds Gathering

You enter your meadow. You are feeling depressed.

As you pass through the gate you settle on the ground on the right hand side of your special space.

As you sit there a dark cloud comes down from up high and settles over and around you.

You are stuck to the spot and can't move in any direction. You can do nothing, say nothing and feel nothing.

You become aware of your breathing. Your breathing, with its inspiration and expiration, is now the centre of your concentration. The breath is everything to you. Your very centre, that which keeps you going and gives you a sense of hope is your breathing. Breathing in and out, in and out brings a wonderful reassurance.

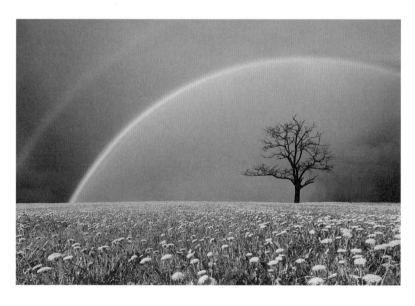

It suddenly starts to rain. It pours down on top of you. There is lightning and thunder. You are soaked to the bone and you are frightened by the ferocity of the storm.

Yet you keep breathing. The breathing with its rhythm, keeps you centred. This is your lowest point — your nadir. But at this moment you can face your dark cloud of depression. You separate from your feelings. You are raised high above them and look down on them like an eagle.

The feelings are still there like a leaden weight but have no power over you as you become a witness to your unhappy feelings. They continue as you look, as you take the active role of observer. You are no longer passive.

As you separate, see, and acknowledge the darkness below, as a sudden change takes place. The clouds around you lift and drift away. The rain, thunder and lightning stops. The sun comes out and a wonderful rainbow arches over your meadow.

You are experiencing the dark and the light. You are living through the swing of the opposites — and you have endured. You see that it was okay to feel the depths of despair but that it is possible to move away from despair and darkness and to not give these feelings power absolutely. You see that it is normal to have these feelings but they can be endured and their power lessened.

You have learned to endure your storm.

Birds now sing and your heart is touched by their beauty. The wind now rushes through the trees and the sound calms your mind. You now see the bright colours of the leaves and flowers. The scents of the nightshade now fill you with a sense of awe.

A little band of musicians dressed in rainbow colours slide down the rainbow. They enter your now bright, shining meadow. They dance around you playing pipes, zithers, bells, bowls, flutes and lutes.

These people are so full of life and joy. They laugh and their songs are full of love. You join with them.

They tell you that they are a special band of players that live deep inside you. They can be called upon at any time. They can help change from one opposite to the other.

These people within you are deeply artistic. They have learned to use the energy within dark depressive clouds and put it into their music. They are also keepers of the colours within plants and the sky, and especially within rainbows.

When you feel the darkness, the dark clouds, know that these musicians are nearby. You know that they are never far away. If you can observe the feelings you will see that there is magic and wonder within this darkness.

You see there is great love, energy and joy within and through despair, if only you can endure and observe. While you watch and be a witness to them the musicians are within gathering energy for the dance of life.

The musicians move back to the rainbow. You lie down in your meadow and pass into a deep sleep, resting deeply because you have endured the opposites and are enriched by their journey from one to the other.

Week 5

Anger to Serenity: Smashing the Rock

You are in your meadow. You are in deep anger. It may be silent anger, passive aggressive, violent anger, rage, explosive anger, mental anger, emotional anger, pressure-cooker anger, white-hot anger, bitterness, hate, loathing, fear or any other sort of anger.

These angers come from the grieving process and are a normal part of recovery.

You see in front of you a large collection of rocks. Beside the rocks are a large range of tools; chisels, hammers and sculpting utensils of all kinds.

By your own hand you begin to shape things.

You understand clearly and immediately that the huge emotions you acknowledge as being present with you want very much to be expressed. These powerful emotions want to live inside a stable form. They long to exist as a form.

They want to be in that rock. They ache for stability.

You listen to these emotions. They are movers and they motivate you with great dynamism. You attack the rock with the tools available to you. With every blow, with every movement you shape. With every scrape you send the energy of anger into the form of the rock.

You begin to see a shape forming.

You scream as you expel these emotions into the rock. There is no one around. There is complete isolation and safety. It is completely up to you whether you dance or sing or scream.

The choice is yours.

After a time you sit exhausted and see that in front of you is a shape. It is your shape, a figure, or simple shape, a cross or a circle or a sphere. It could be a fountain or an animal shape. It can be a shape or form never seen before.

You sit and admire the shaped rock. Your anger is gone and now exists in front of you. You feel great peace and serenity. The

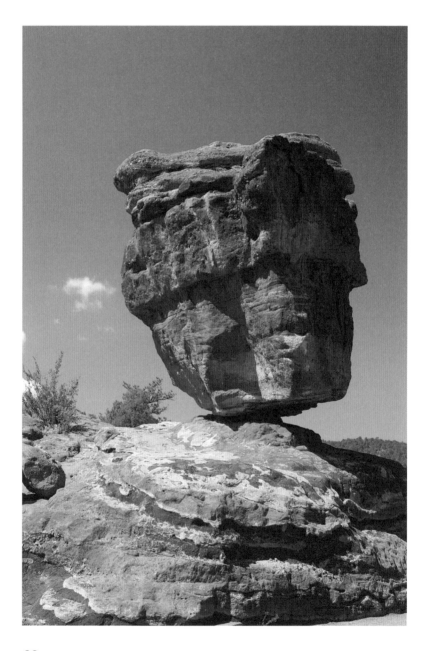

anger itself is now solid and secure. It has found a form and is now secure. You are no longer the place where it resides.

The anger has helped you be creative. This beautiful sculpture now resides in a special place in your meadow.

The sun falls down on the new creation and it glitters and sparkles in the light.

You fall into a deep slumber. You rest deeply and feel satisfied and healed.

Your heart is now filled with your flame burning and you see a soft red colour in your heart.

There is wonderful warmth in your chest area.

When you awake you feel energised and calm within your very core. You leave the meadow and take these feelings with you.

Week 6

Self Doubt to Confidence: The Little Self and the Big Self

You are heading towards your meadow. You walk slowly because you are swamped with a feeling of self-doubt.

You come to the gate of your meadow but are slow to enter. You feel not worthy of being in such a beautiful place.

It takes ages to find the key to enter.

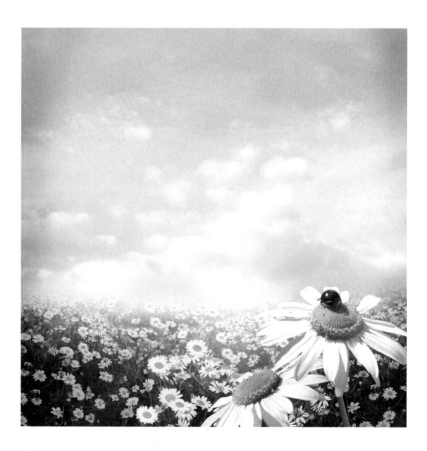

When you manage to enter you slump to the ground. You then find that you have become very small. You see alongside you a scarab beetle and realise you are the same size. An ant passes by and you look at it in the eye.

At this stage down at that level even the grass seems like a rainforest. It is large and extremely difficult to move through. It becomes dark, dank and claustrophobic.

You enter the state of the little self. You are so small that even normal small things become big and overwhelming.

You are in the state called self-doubt. You cannot move forward or back; you are immobilised, everything seems too big and threatening.

You ask for help and it comes immediately.

Help is in the shape of a big bumble bee. It is busy pollinating flowers but sees you hiding behind a tiny leaf.

The bee asks you why you are so small today, and says that as owner of the meadow you are normally walking tall.

As you hear this and are reminded of your splendid inheritance you grow a little bit bigger.

As you begin to be more mobile you stumble a little further. You can now put your head above the grass. As you do so you are greeted by a butterfly who asks what is wrong with you. "You are normally so much bigger," says the beautiful butterfly.

This reminds you again of your inheritance which you have recently rediscovered and you again grow slightly bigger.

Then you come across an army of ants. They surround you in a circle and one, their leader, steps forward to speak to you.

He says that he, along with the beetles, butterflies, animals and insects, live here in your meadow. He says that you are much valued and loved. He says that this is your meadow and that they all work for the common good. You are the centre of the meadow and without your ordering and maintenance it would fall into ruin. "We need you and you need us."

You are filled with confidence and feel very much part of

the place. You see that you, the place, its plants and animals and insects are all one, and that you are very much part of that oneness.

You grow tall again. You grow big by being part of the whole.

Your own self-centred view of yourself had made you small. The little-self is you, separate and full of ideas about yourself.

The big-self is the all. Being a part of it all brings confidence and strength.

You drift off to sleep. You are embraced by all around you — by the big-self.

Week 7

Hate to Love: The String and the Heart

You are walking nearby to your meadow but are not yet inside its boundaries.

You realise that you have an uncomfortable feeling of hate within you. You look down on the emotion inside you. You observe it, without judgement.

The hate then becomes a big black coat and you find yourself wearing it.

The coat has many pockets associated with this negative emotion. Each pocket is filled with other relatives of hate; loathing, cynicism, sarcasm, irritability, justification, moodiness, depression, illness, lack of energy, sourness, revenge and many others.

You enter through your gate into your special space. The coat

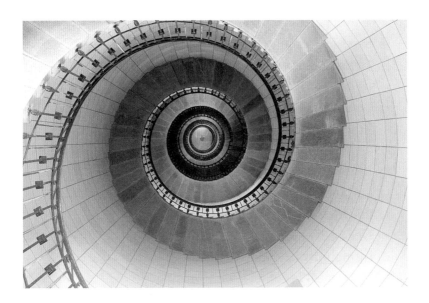

hangs heavy with all these emotions and you walk slowly. You drag yourself along.

As you walk into your meadow, you see a huge shining spiral. It is made out of a very long piece of woven string. It has a silver appearance.

You can make out little bits of something on the weave but at this stage you don't know exactly what it is made of.

You start to walk to walk around the spiral which reaches up into the sky. You reach into one of your many pockets and take out one of the many anger associated states. The states have all turned, in the depth of the pockets into a black gooey substance. You take this sticky state, the first one being pure hate, and throw it into the spirally energy in front of you and above you.

As you do this a beautiful gemstone, a deep red ruby ring falls to the ground. You take it and put it on.

As you put the ruby ring on your finger you find that you can step onto the spiral. You then begin to walk up the spiral. You feel safe and secure doing this.

As you walk up the spiral you empty each pocket, of the many pockets, and fling the dark emotions upwards.

Each emotion you throw is replaced in the pocket from which it came by a precious stone:

- Sarcasm becomes a topaz.
- Cynicism becomes a black opal.
- Irritability becomes a citrine.
- Justification becomes an aquamarine.
- Moodiness becomes a blue topaz.
- Depression becomes an emerald.
- Illness becomes a lapis lazuli.
- Lack of energy becomes an amethyst.
- Sourness becomes a black pearl.
- Negativity becomes a garnet.
- Immobility becomes a sapphire.
- Unfairness becomes a white opal.

- Revenge becomes a bloodstone.
- Powerlessness becomes a moonstone.

The coat now turns into a light and beautiful one. It is now shining with all the colours of the gemstones.

Your body is warm. The red from your ruby ring glows and a red colour enters your heart. You feel warmth inside you.

Whenever you think of the ruby and its precious sister stones and the black pearl you think of the transformation of dark things into objects that catch the light.

- You see that hate can be turned to love.
- Cynicism can be turned into wellbeing.
- Sarcasm can be turned into peace.
- Irritability can be turned into harmony.
- Justification can be turned into fun.
- Moodiness can be turned into use.
- Illness can be turned into wellness.
- Depression can be turned into hope.
- Lethargy can be turned into energy.
- Sourness can be turned into beauty.
- Negativity can be turned into possibilities.
- Immobility can be turned into movement.
- Unfairness can be turned into fairness.
- Revenge can be turned into compassion.
- Powerlessness can be turned into conscious passivity.

You now find yourself back in your meadow. You lie on the grass still wearing your coat. As you drift off to sleep the coat dissolves and enters into your being as a bright and shining rainbow coloured light.

When you awake you find some beautiful coloured stones beside you on the grass. You take them with you as you walk through your gate and out of your meadow.

Week 8

Weakness to Strength: The Mouse and the Bear

You are outside your meadow.

You are filled with weakness. You shiver with an unpleasant lack of substance. You are pale and thin inside. You quiver and apologise for yourself (even though there is no one else there.)

You enter through your gate and go into your meadow so that you can, in safety, explore this unpleasant state.

You huddle into a corner somewhere and weep and shudder at having to face the world.

After a while you lift your head and see in front of you a little field mouse. He is wearing bright colours and has a tennis racquet in his hands. He asks what the trouble is. You gather yourself and tell him that you have been feeling poorly lately and that you don't know what to do with yourself.

He asks you whether you realise that within your secret place, the meadow, there was an even more secret place. You say no and he asks whether he can take you there. He says that there is something important for you there.

You say yes and he scurries away and you follow him. You go through some dales and through a wooded part and past a stream and then into a slightly rocky place. You follow as he takes you into a huge cave which dips down at the back into a small passage and out into a really big space.

In the space a meeting is going on. There are about one hundred seats. On the seats are mice and other related rodents. They are all sitting in their seats looking small, fearful and anxious. You sit in a seat with your name on it. You have shrunk so that you are almost as small as the mice.

In front of this meeting of mice and rodents is a huge brown bear.

He sits and reads a recipe marked 'Courage Mixture'. It is a recipe known only to bears. Bears are the holders of courage. He bellows out orders to those around him. He is very strong.

There is a big pot with a fire underneath brewing on the stage. There is a beautiful smell of the forest coming from the brew.

The helper mice throw some pine cones into the mixture.

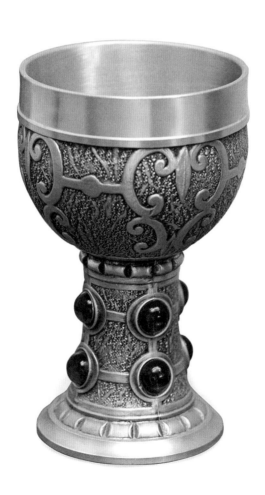

Honey is dropped into the brew by some hard working bees.

More mice add special herbs and leaves from the courage tree.

When the brew is ready a queue forms at the right of the stage. Your friend the mouse urges you to join the queue.

Each little animal takes a tiny silver chalice and is given a small amount of courage fluid.

You take yours and you sit back on your seat. Your heart fills with a strength that you have never felt before. You feel a steel presence in your heart.

You look into your heart and see a huge bear. It stays with you as you walk out of the meeting. You look around. Each little animal has a strong look in their eyes regardless of how small they are physically.

You walk back; your tiny friend is scurrying ahead practising his tennis shots. You then return to the centre of your meadow. Before he scurries off he says to call on him when you need to fill up with some more courage fluid. He will always appear when you grow small again.

When you grow small again the mouse says he will automatically come to you and take you to the secret bear place to attend another meeting to drink the bear's special brew.

Week 9

Terror to Calm: The Storm on the Lake

You are about to enter your meadow. You take another state which you can safely explore in this special place. It is terror — extreme fear.

This is a perfectly normal part of the grieving process. You can now safely be a witness to it. You feel safe to examine these things in your meadow.

It is evening and you go through the gate of your special place. You feel an extreme anxiety welling up in your heart. You are in a precarious situation.

You see something new in this space. In the middle of your land is a large stretch of water. It shimmers in the dusky light.

In the middle of the lake is an island.

You get an urge to get to the island. You sense that there is safety there.

You see a little row boat on the edge of the water.

You start to row.

As you make progress a storm quickly emerges. Dark clouds gather.

Lightning cuts through the air. Thunder makes a bone-penetrating sound.

Rain pours down on top of you. The temperature drops. The water is choppy and dangerous. Your boat is thrown around in dangerous swells as the strong wind churns up big waves on the lake's surface.

You are extremely threatened and frightened.

Your terror within is manifesting outside. Your inner storm, the one you are now seeing, is a storm outside of you.

You have no torch, no weather equipment, and no life-jacket. The boat is thrown around. You are helpless. You start to panic. You can no longer see the island which promised so much.

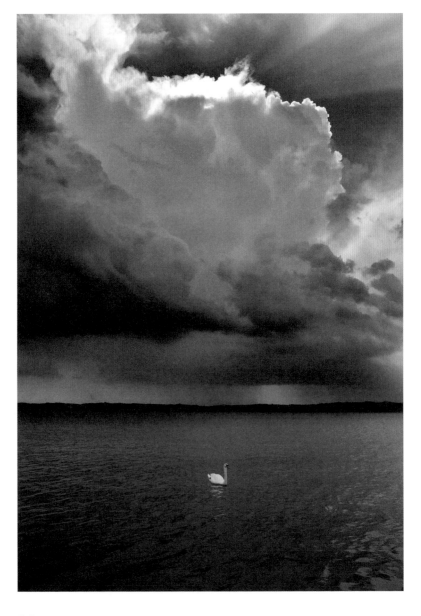

You are in the dark. You can't see a way out.

However, you do see one thing that brings hope.

You see a dim light in the distance. You muster your strength to move towards the light. You work hard. You endure. This struggle is long and hard. You give it all you've got.

You let the terror go as you struggle. You aim to get to the light, to a calmer place. You let go of the terror as you work. You put all your energy into getting to safety. Your anxiety fades because you have no time or place for it. It impedes your struggle. You let it go.

You feel the storm lessening. You feel stronger. Hope begins to fill your heart. You feel as though there is now a way out. You are fighting. You are exhilarated by your progress. You are now in control of your own destiny. This begins to feel good as you are empowered by your wonderful determination.

Anxiety and terror are replaced by effort and self-determination. You are doing all you can and now you fate is in *your* hands. You struggle as hard as you can and you, knowing this, accept the outcome — in peace.

As you see this you sight land in front of you. It is the island in the middle of the water.

You get out of the boat. You walk towards the middle of the island.

You see a tiny hut above and walk to it. It is a simple hut. You enter.

In the hut a fire burns. You see a towel and a change of clothes. You dry yourself and get into the fresh white clothes. You sit before the fire in a comfortable armchair. You feel at ease.

You look out the window and see that the storm has stopped. The calm outside reflects your new inner state.

The terror, through the struggle, has become calm.

You see a dove which flies onto the window sill.

You fall asleep to the cooing of the dove knowing that in the morning you will return to your meadow over calm waters.

You will then leave through the gate and go home in a new state knowing that when you struggle through a future storm the island and its simple wooden hut is there to receive you, warm you and give you protection and solace.

Week 10

The Wonderful Conclusion

You now start to look back on your wonderful journey. You arrive in your meadow and see that there is a new irrigation system at work. It is watering your wonderful new garden.

The water from the sprinklers has a grey colour about it. It is grey water.

This water has a compost sort of smell. It is full of your fear, pain, depression, anger, self-doubt, hate, weakness and terror. All these things have been transformed in you and you can now use them as fertiliser on your inner garden. They have been witnessed, brought into the light, broken down, and liquefied into mulch.

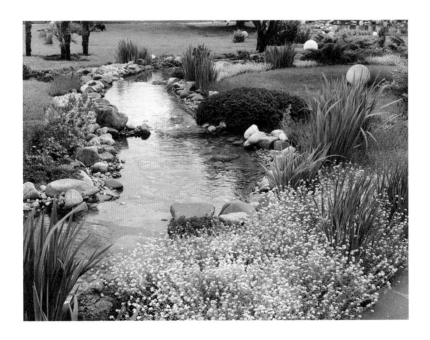

These waste products can now be used for your garden's growth.

You now see that there's a gathering in front of you of some special helpers. There are five male helpers and five female helpers.

The first is a boy of around ten. He represents carefree happiness. This is a mental state.

The second is a man of twenty. He represents strength. This is a physical state.

The third is a man of thirty. He represents love. This is an emotional state.

The fourth is a man of fifty. He represents confidence. This is a psychological state.

The fifth is a man of eighty. He represents serenity. This is a spiritual state.

The sixth is a girl of twelve. She represents happiness. This is an emotional state.

The seventh is a woman of twenty-five. She represents confidence. This is a mental state.

The eighth is a woman of thirty-nine. She represents calm. This is a physical state.

The ninth is a woman of fifty-five. She represents strength. This is a psychological state.

The tenth is a woman of eighty-three. She represents serenity. This is a spiritual state.

These are states of womanhood and manhood.

They all stand in front of you. They each bring a different element and skill to build your garden.

You send them to work. You use your intuition and perception to see what task they do.

You are taught by what task you see that they each do.

They form a circle around you. You are at the centre of this circle.

The circle moves in a clockwise direction.

As it turns it enters you. The circle enters and goes deep inside you. It rotates in your heart.

You feel a deep healing taking place. These people go to their appropriate place. They are healers and they begin to heal. They take their place and begin to heal you. They move through your body doing their tasks.

You can speak to these healers and ask where they are and what they are working on. You start a journal with the conversations you have with them.

You feel your inner garden being worked on. It is fertilised by the new irrigation and cultivated by these workers. They tend your garden permanently.

Your garden becomes richer, more fertile and more beautiful the more that you do these exercises.

You can return to your garden any time to repeat any of these exercises. The garden becomes richer and more rewarding each time you go.

The Journey of the Stones

Week 1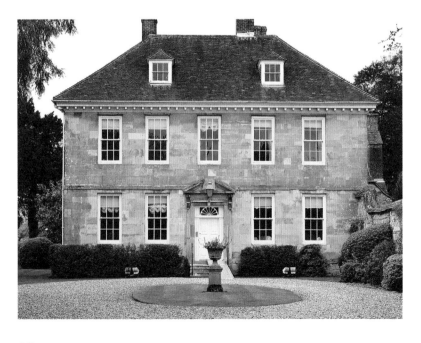

The Immune System:
Dalmatian Stone and The Wishing Well

About the Dalmatian Stone

Physical characteristics: Pale yellow with black specks, a bit like the specks on a Dalmatian dog.

Chakra: It is associated with the base and solar plexus chakras.

Metaphysical qualities: It is believed to be a stone of strength, one that helps people overcome being overly analytical and move towards a life filled with fun and forward movement. It helps people find their true purpose in life.

Effect on the body: Physically it works on breaking down things in the same way digestion breaks down food and the intestines help break down gallstones.

The meditation

Take time to relax and lie down. Breathe deeply for a few minutes placing the stone on your chest. Close your eyes.

See yourself walking in a country place; walk down safe and familiar tracks and hear the sound of birds and frogs. You see small animals, flowering bushes and the beautiful play of light on the greenery around you.

You come to an old house. At the entrance there are huge iron gates. The gates are opened by an old gardener who is accompanied by a housekeeper. They embrace you with warmth and love. They say that they have been expecting you. They say that they have hidden ten stones on the property. These are stones of self-discovery and healing, and you must find all ten to fully strengthen yourself. The first stone is hidden in the garden and as you walk through you see bees on flowers, ants on the ground, the bark on trees and palms in the conservatory.

You walk around to the back of the building and you see a grotto. It is here that a wonderful sense of peace comes over you. You sit by the water's edge and you see your reflection. You see that there is a shiny object at the bottom of the pool. As you look closer you see the Dalmatian stone. You pick it up and hold it and all the wonderful memories of your life return to you.

You might see:

- A day at the beach.
- The birth of a child.
- A first meeting.
- A time of peace.
- A moment of love.
- A sunrise.
- Holding a beloved animal.

- ‣ All personal achievements.
- ‣ Other positive memories.

The energy of these positive recalls floods through your body and fills it with a bright shiny light. It wells around and enters your immune system filling it with stores of energy. Golden light floods through your vitals. You feel strong reinforced and healthy.

Placing the stone back in the grotto pool you make a wish.

The gardener and housekeeper, your protectors, have made a wonderful afternoon tea in the garden for you.

After you leave through the gate you find yourself in the country lane.

Take five minutes to breathe slowly and then return to the present moment and then move the body slowly before returning to a sitting position.

Week 2

The Nervous System:
Mahogany Stone and the Circle Of Support

About the Mahogany Stone
Physical characteristics: This obsidian stone is a natural volcanic glass which has a reddish brown matrix with splashes of black colour. It was used in the Stone Age to make tools and also as an ornamental stone.

Chakra: It balances the first chakra and is grounding.

Metaphysical qualities: It provides strength in times of need. It facilitates fulfilment of life aspirations, eliminates energy blocks and relieves tension. It promotes a forgiving attitude and releases grievances. It is sometimes called the mirror stone because it reflects one's shortcomings that are dealt with then let go. It is believed to help with decision making.

Effect on the body: It removes pain and improves circulation.

The meditation
Lie down on your mat; breathe deeply for a few minutes.

You are back walking in your country lane. You feel relaxed and calm looking around at the beautiful scenery. You come to your wonderful old house.

Your two carers are waiting for you and you enter through the gate. They tell you that the second stone is hidden in an earthy place.

As you start to look you walk past the stables, fruit trees, chook pens and empty herb beds.

Sniffing the air you are greeted with a strong smell which

comes from a big compost heap. You know that your stone is at the bottom of it so you start to dig and you move the compost onto the empty herb bed. You find your stone and also a box of seeds. You plant the seeds in the bed and then water it. You

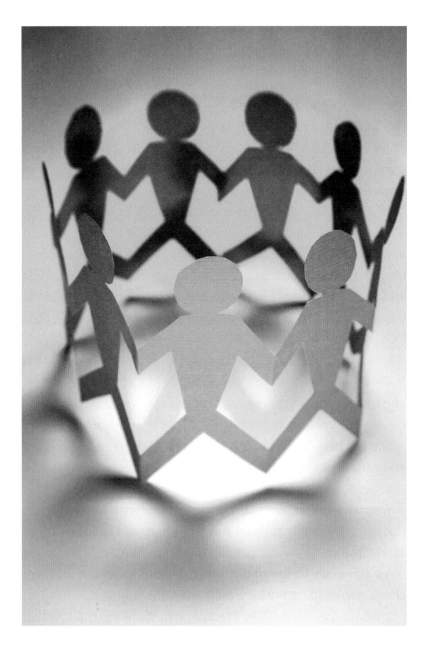

then sit down in front of it on some grass. You place the stone on your sacral area. The energy enters your nervous system.

- ▸ You begin to see several people who have thought highly of you over your life. These people might be: friends, coaches, work colleagues, local shopkeepers, teachers, religious figures, family members, lovers, admirers or others.

These people have admired you and they form a circle of support around you — you feel respected and acknowledged. They take you into their heart.

At this point the elders have arrived and have set up another afternoon tea and your guests join in the celebration.

After this you leave by the iron gates and return to the country lane feeling supported deep inside you.

You breathe deeply on your mat for a few minutes before rising.

Week 3

The Digestive System:
Nephrite Jade and the Little People

About the Nephrite Jade
Physical characteristics: It ranges from dark green, which is rich in iron, to a creamy colour, which means the stone has a high magnesium content. Nephrite jade may be homogeneous in colour, banded or blotchy.

Chakra: It is the heart chakra so has a beneficial effect on all love relationships.

Metaphysical qualities: It is considered to be good for emotional balance and stability. It is a protective stone and with energetic clearing properties. In Chinese tradition, jade symbolised the five virtues of humanity: wisdom, compassion, justice, modesty and courage. Symbols of these virtues were often carved into jade.

Effect on the body: It is often used in the crystal healing of the physical heart, and kidney problems.

The meditation
Lie down on your mat with your eyes closed, breathing deeply for a few minutes.

You are once again in your beautiful country lane outside the iron gates of your special house. The elders are there to welcome you.

You start walking and looking for your stone. You go past the grotto and see the compost heap. You look at the grass and see ants, bees, ladybirds, grasshoppers and also fish in the pond.

You then see a big herb garden, full of hundreds of different types of herbs. As you look into the garden you see a hundred herbs moving and dancing exchanging great energies and smells. It is a living mass of healing power.

You sit in front of it and feel the great energy.

In the middle of the herb garden is a country-style pale green chair. Shining in the middle of the chair is your nephrite jade stone.

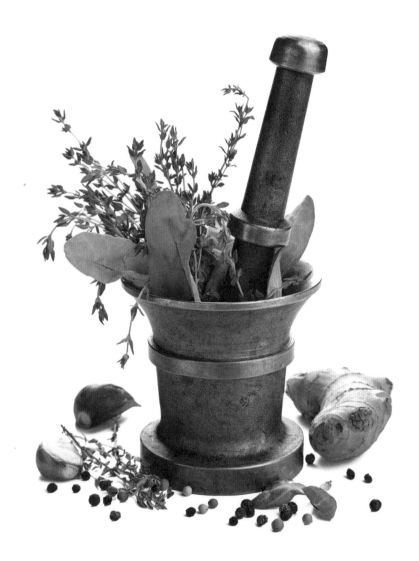

You walk to the garden chair and sit down, placing the stone on your stomach. As you focus you see seven garden spirits, male and female, gather in front of the waving green herbs. They smile at you and say that they love you and haven't seen you since you were a child. They say that they have something for you that will make you feel strong and invulnerable, full of green energy and healing. One at a time they disappear and re-emerge with a glass thimble of green juice extracted from the herbs. They range from light pale green to dark, black green. You drink each thimbleful in turn.

This potent liquid passes into your digestive system cleansing, restoring and energising. You feel powerful and renewed.

The two elders have made a wonderful afternoon tea. The seven little people join in the fun.

Week 4

The Circulatory System:
The Bloodstone and the Purity Tree

About the Bloodstone (Heliotrope)

Physical characteristics: It is dark green with distinctive red spots that resemble blood. The red spots are due to the presence of iron oxides in the mineral. The legend of the origin of bloodstone says that it was first formed when some drops of Christ's blood fell and stained some jasper at the foot of the cross.

Chakra: It is associated with root and heart chakras.

Metaphysical properties: In ancient folklore, bloodstone was said to give off audible sounds as a guide. It gives one the

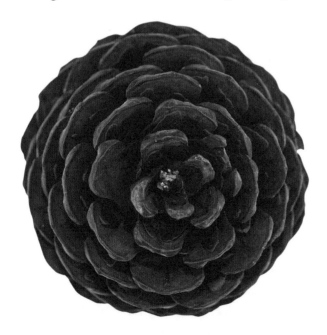

ability to banish evil and negativity of all kinds. The Greeks and Romans wore bloodstone for endurance during athletic endeavours and to secure favour of those in power. The later Gnostics believed that this stone prolonged life and brought untold wealth.

Effect on the body: Bloodstone is used to aid in circulation of all energy in the body and helps to remove energy blocks. Some believe it cleanses the blood, stimulates the immune system to fight infections and detoxifies. Ancient Egyptians used bloodstone to treat tumours.

The meditation

Lie down on your mat with your eyes closed and breathe deeply for five minutes.

You are walking in your country lane. You enter through the iron gates. You are welcomed by your elders. You start to walk and look for stones. You go past the grotto, the compost heap and the herb garden.

You look up into a huge pine tree, with its thick trunk, needles, and leaves, and beyond into the blue sky.

A pine cone falls at your feet. You pick it up and it turns into a bloodstone. You stand in front of the tree and a strange thing happens; when you squeeze the stone you are able to sense the tree and its life and movement, but when you release the squeeze you are able to sense the life and circulation within yourself.

You squeeze and enter the circulatory system of the tree and water surges upwards through the roots. Sap surges through the multiple highways of the trunk and out into branches, leaves and pine cones. Sunlight is taken in and there is a huge transformation of energies. These then move back down the trunk, round and round like a huge blood system. Leaves and cones are produced creating profound energies.

You squeeze and feel your own circulation system. You squeeze twice and a remarkable thing happens. The energy of the tree passes into the bloodstone which is placed on your heart chakra and joins with your own circulatory system.

This energy cleans and purifies. It travels through you into the ground and is taken up by the tree. A great circular miracle takes place.

You feel powerful and strong. You blood is richer, cleaner and more purified. This new circulation cleanses your body of disease and nothing can hurt you now.

You gather with your elders who have made a wonderful afternoon tea under the shade of the tree.

You leave through the iron gates and find yourself in the country lane.

Take some time to breathe with your eyes closed before getting off your mat.

Week 5

The Heart and Lungs:
Crazy Lace Agate and the Loving Embrace

About the Crazy Blue Lace Agate Stone

Physical characteristics: Blue lace agate is a banded variety of chalcedony. It is a pale blue stone, with delicate white banding.

Chakra: It is associated with the throat chakra.

Metaphysical properties: A very cooling and calming stone, which promotes a sense of peace and tranquillity. A powerful throat healer, it assists with the verbal expression of thoughts and feelings. It nurtures, supports, neutralises anger, infection, inflammation and fever.

Effect on the body: It is believed to strengthen and accelerate the repair of bones, thyroid deficiencies, and throat and lymph infections. It soothes sore eyes and skin problems associated with redness and irritation.

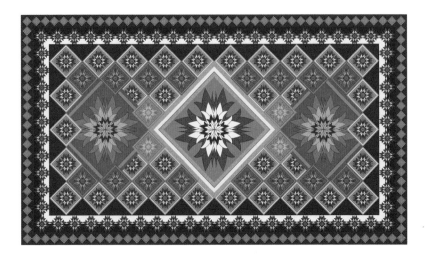

The meditation

Lie down on your mat; breathe slowly for a few minutes with your eyes closed.

You are walking down your beautiful country lane. Your elders greet you at the iron gates. They tell you to look for your stone in an elevated place.

You walk towards the house looking at the balconies and find a roof garden with a spiral staircase leading up to it.

At the top of the garden there is a beautiful Persian carpet. Lying on top of this is your crazy lace agate stone sparkling in the sun. You lie down on the carpet placing the stone on the crown of your head. You look up and examine the blue of the sky and breathe deeply for a few minutes. You feel the top of your head open and expand into the sky and beyond. You become all the planets and stars, the solar system and the universe.

You stay expanded like this for a few minutes. You then slowly bring yourself back from the universe, solar system, Milky Way, planets and stars until it is just you and the blue sky again.

The beautiful blue sky colour enters through the top of your head and is brought into your lungs. This brings deep peace. You feel the lungs embrace the heart. Your heart is a deep red colour. It feels protected by the lungs and the lungs feel deeply loved by the heart. Take the red through each cell of the body. Each cell becomes a tiny outpost of this love and has within a tiny red heart. You feel energised and powerful. You spread this love through the house and down into the garden where your elders are waiting for you with a wonderful afternoon tea.

You leave through the iron gates and find yourself in the country lane feeling empowered and enthusiastic with life.

You take five minutes sitting on your mat before opening your eyes.

Week 6

The Spinal Column:
White Onyx and the Resting Place

About the White Onyx Stone

Physical characteristics: The white onyx usually has alternating light and dark bands, which are coloured brown, red, black, white and grey. Onyx is often recommended to athletes as it is believed to increase strength, endurance, perseverance, and explosiveness, especially if placed on the solar plexus.

Chakra: White onyx is connected to the first chakra, muladhara, and is believed to link this base or root chakra to the crown chakra, creating balanced energy throughout the chakra system.

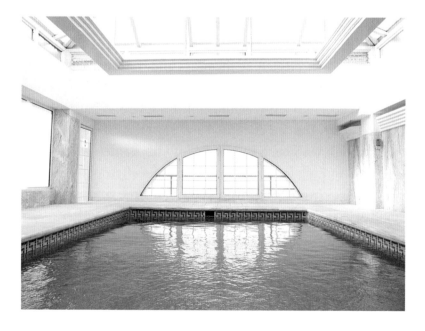

Metaphysical qualities: White onyx is good for releasing negative emotions such as sorrow and grief. It is also believed to bring good fortune and help people recognise their own personal strength. It also helps with relaxation, and in facing various challenges in life, especially a lack of life energy and exhaustion.

Effect on the body: Onyx has been used in the treatment of disorders in the bone marrow, feet and soft tissues of the body.

The meditation

Lie down on your mat and breathe slowly for a few minutes with your eyes closed.

You are walking down your beautiful country lane. Your elders greet you at the iron gates. They tell you that the white onyx is in the shining place.

You walk through the garden and round the house, by the grotto, compost garden, herb garden, big tree, circular staircase and roof garden and back through the laundry, kitchen and pantry where you find a white door that leads to the bathing room.

This is a big room with black and white floor tiles and in the centre a large sunken pool. You take off your clothes and swim to the middle of the pool. You see the stone shining at the bottom. You retrieve the stone and swim to the side of the pool. You place your head in a headrest.

You place the stone on your forehead. A skylight opens in the ceiling above you and a white light enters your forehead through the stone and travels down your spinal column.

All pain and negativity are removed and you feel a deep sense of relaxation. A state of bliss moves through all the cells of the body. You release pain, negativity, depression and anxiety into the warm bath water.

A white light enters the pool and dispenses all the sadness, pain and self-doubt that you have released into the waters.

You float in a place of peace and tranquillity, you feel warm and supported.

You get out of the pool leaving the stone in the water so it is always there when you need it.

You put on some beautiful white linen clothes and rose oil. When you are dressed the elders join you for a wonderful afternoon tea.

You leave through the iron gates and find yourself in the country lane with a wonderful feeling of peace which stays with you for a long time.

You take five minutes sitting on your mat before opening your eyes.

Week 7

The Kidneys:
Carnelian and the Gift of the Bees

About the Carnelian Stone

Physical characteristics: The carnelian stone is a translucent, reddish orange. The various shades of red are due to the presence of iron oxide. Stones may be uniformly coloured or faintly banded. The best carnelian is from India, where it is placed in the sun to change from brown to various shades of red.

Chakra: It is associated with the second or navel chakra.

Metaphysical qualities: It aids in understanding the inner self and strengthens concentration. Some ancient cultures believed

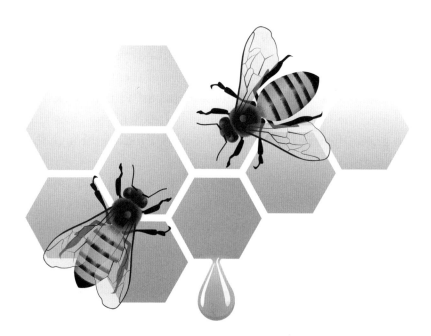

the carnelian offered protection during travels after death and against evil.

Effect on the body: It was once thought to still the blood and calm the temper. It is believed to increase self-esteem and stimulate creativity. It dispels negative energies and replaces them with positive ones.

The meditation

Lie down on your mat; breathe slowly for a few minutes with your eyes closed.

You are walking down your beautiful country lane. Your elders greet you at the iron gates.

They tell you to look for the stone in the 'golden place'. You start to walk around to the back of the house and in the distance you see an old man, the beekeeper, who is attending to his hives. He is a kind and caring man who loves his bees. He says to you that the bees know you from childhood and have been waiting for you to return. He says that they have a beautiful gift for you.

The beekeeper then places a big piece of honeycomb onto a nearby table and this turns into the carnelian stone.

You rub the stone over your lower back and over your kidneys.

You look over at the bees and twelve of them fly off in the direction of the woods. You follow them past a small forest into an area the size of a meadow. It is barren with no trees and no grass. There is a smelly, derelict creek running through the property.

The twelve bees turn into twelve young men and women. They begin to work on a wonderful project of renewal.

You join them — trees are planted, the creek is cleaned and freed up, native bush tucker plants and grasses are sown, strong undergrowth is planted for stability.

You hold the stone in your hand and can see into the future. You see birds have returned and are nesting, insects and small animals now live in comfort and peace, trees are laden with fruit, the creek is flowing, small fish and frogs have returned, and dragonflies skit over the water's surface.

As you look at this wonderful scene the twelve bees return, buzzing with pleasure around the garden.

The two elders have returned with a wonderful afternoon tea.

You leave through the iron gates and find yourself in the country lane with a wonderful feeling of peace which stays with you for a long time.

You take five minutes sitting on your mat before opening your eyes.

Week 8

The Skeletal System:
African Turquoise and the Talking Books

About the Green African Turquoise Stone

Physical characteristics: African turquoise is a type of spotted teal jasper rather than turquoise.

Chakra: It is associated with the fourth chakra and self acceptance.

Metaphysical qualities: Some spiritualists believe that African turquoise will attract money to the wearer. It is also believed by some to offer protection from accidents while travelling. Emotionally, some think that African turquoise will encourage self-trust. It is also thought to allow the wearer to express themselves more clearly.

Effect on body: It is believed to reduce headaches.

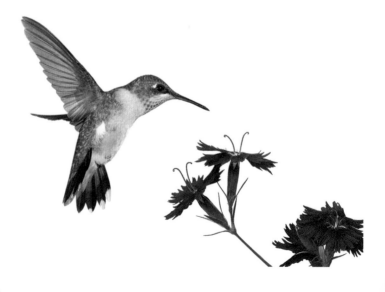

The meditation

Lie down on your mat; breathe slowly for a few minutes with your eyes closed.

You are walking down your beautiful country lane. Your elders greet you at the iron gates.

The elders say that your stone is waiting for you in the clever corner. You start to walk, by the grotto, compost garden, herb garden, big tree, circular staircase pool and roof hives. You go into the house and look around. You go upstairs through several rooms and then into a big library.

In the corner a beautiful stone is sitting on a little roll-top desk. You walk over and sit at the desk placing the stone on your sternum.

A light from your stone marks a book on the shelf entitled *Love*. You get the book, take it to the desk and open it.

You see several images:

- Two people walking hand in hand on a beach.
- A child with an animal.
- A bird feeding its young.
- Beautiful spring flowers.
- A mother with her child.

You turn to page two and see several of your own images. These wonderful images fill you with love and joy. You let this feeling flow into the marrow of your bones.

You see the light from your stone catch another book called *Beauty*. You open the first page and see:

- A flower opening slowly.
- A beautiful sunset.
- A fabulous sunrise.
- A humming bird drinking nectar.
- A valley full of emerging monarch butterflies.

You open page two and you see your own images of beauty. You let these images flow into the skeletal system.

The light then sets on another book called *Compassion*. You open page one and see:

- A deaf child hearing for the first time.
- A foal being born.
- The breaking of drought.
- Someone saying "sorry".
- A community caring for others that need help.

You open page two and see your own acts of compassion. You take this feeling through every bone in your body.

You then walk down into the garden where your elders are waiting for you with a wonderful afternoon tea.

You leave through the iron gates and find yourself in the country lane with a wonderful feeling of deep love in your heart. This feeling stays with you for a long time.

You take five minutes sitting on your mat before opening your eyes.

Week 9

The Thyroid Gland: Blue Quartz and the Wonderful Marriage

About the Blue Quartz (Dumortierite) Stone

Physical characteristics: The blue quartz is a man-made stone. It is usually pale to medium blue with very small tourmaline that reflect blue light.

Chakra: It is associated with the fifth chakra, the throat chakra. It balances the throat chakra and enhances communication between the lower chakras (physical realm) and the high chakras (in the spiritual realm). It is also associated with the seventh chakra, the third eye chakra.

Metaphysical qualities: Quartz is one of the seven precious substances of Buddhism. It releases fear and brings courage to one's life. It boosts creativity and expression. Ancient priests used quartz crystals to render negative energy impotent, to dissolve enchantments, spells and destroy all black magic.

Effect on the body: The Romans used quartz for glandular swelling, fevers and as a pain reliever. In Medieval times quartz was held against the tongue to assuage fever and quench thirst. Scottish Highland quartz set in silver and worn on the back was said to be effective for kidney disease.

The meditation

Lie down on your mat; breathe slowly for a few minutes with your eyes closed.

You are walking down your beautiful country lane. Your elders greet you at the iron gates.

They tell you that your stone is in a place of learning. You start to walk by the grotto, the compost heap, the herb garden, a big tree, circular staircase, the pool and the hives. You go into the house and look around. You enter the house and walk through several rooms until you find the study. This is big room with pleasant lighting, shelves and a large desk.

You see the stone shining on the desktop. You hold it to your throat and as you do this a scene appears before you. You go deep into your heart and your deepest wishes come up on the screen. This is now out of your control but you trust the process and let the images flow. You see pictures of what you want, what you think, what you feel, and what you really need to do.

For example, you might see yourself writing books, journals, or letters. You might see yourself drawing, painting, sculpting or taking photographs. You might see yourself playing cards

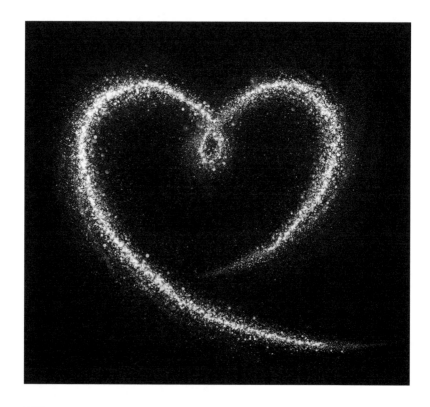

with people, going for walks, organising outings, going to the cinema, the museum, a gallery or the library. You might see yourself listening to lectures, going to a course, or learning a new language. You might see yourself making new friends, seeing old friends, going to church or travelling. You might see yourself gardening or participating in bush regeneration. You might see yourself joining in on a cooking course or reading groups.

You only see things on the screen connected with your love.

Now you see on the screen a planning diary — daily, monthly and yearly. You organise your time and a list of your goals. You see your new schedule comes from deep within you with order, variety and clarity.

You heart and these new plans merge and you feel great strength from the marriage of heart and mind. The energy of love and order enters the stone on your throat. It fills your thyroid gland with golden energy.

You then walk down into the garden where your elders are waiting for you with a wonderful afternoon tea.

You leave through the iron gates and find yourself in the country lane with a wonderful feeling of deep love in your heart, which stays with you for a long time.

You take five minutes sitting on your mat before opening your eyes.

Week 10

The Whole Body:
Peach Aventine and Deep Space

About the Peach Aventine Stone

Physical characteristics: Peach aventine is a light orange colour, sometimes verging on red. Silver flecks are sometimes present and these are believed to help channel healing energy from mother earth to the body.

Chakra: It is associated with the sacral chakra.

Energetic qualities: It helps with shyness and anxiety. It builds confidence, providing dignity, presence and calm. It helps with decision making and can boost creativity. It is sometimes referred to as the 'whisper stone'.

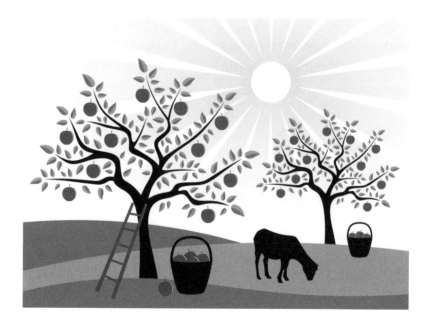

Effect on the body: It is beneficial for the lungs, heart, adrenal glands, the urinary system, and the female reproductive organs, particularly the ovaries.

The meditation

Lie down on your mat; breathe slowly for a few minutes with your eyes closed.

You are walking down your beautiful country lane. Your elders greet you at the iron gates.

You walk to the top of the house and find a room with a circular shape made of glass. The peach aventine stone is on a small table next to a huge telescope. You hold the stone in your hand and look through the telescope into space. You see a huge body of people spread over a huge meeting room. These people mix with a feeling of peace and harmony. They all know each other and they all eat, drink and enjoy themselves.

There is beautiful music and a flowing fountain. Filtered light crosses the room.

You focus on a group to your left; they are the 'grotto group'. These are people associated with wonderful moments of your life.

The second group are the people from the circle of support.

The third group are little people with trays of green drinks and cakes.

The fourth group have a beam of golden light that brings joy to all that they speak to.

The fifth group with blue lungs and red hearts and a loving embrace.

The sixth group have a white light that comes from above and sprinkles down like a soft rain.

The seventh group has a bee at a honey table giving people tiny glasses of honey.

The eighth group are all people from the 'talking books' scenes.

The ninth group all have their hearts and minds working as one.

You see that they are all part of your body, mind and spirit all working together.

You see your elders. They bring you back down to the garden. They hug and embrace you and tell you how much they love you and respect you. They have prepared a wonderful afternoon for you.

As you leave through the iron gates and find yourself in the country lane with a wonderful feeling of deep love in your heart, which stays with you for a long time.

You take five minutes sitting on your mat before opening your eyes.

PART 4

Personal Stories

Becoming a Human Being rather than a Human Doing

Dr Lyn Gow

I offered to write a chapter for this book because I felt that there was so much to write about the journey I have travelled this past year since being diagnosed with breast cancer. The diagnosis was followed rather quickly by a bilateral mastectomy, six rounds of heavy-duty chemotherapy, six weeks of radiation and then ongoing medication to block oestrogen production which was found to have contributed significantly to my diagnosis. The year has witnessed a steep and fascinating learning curve as I had to make ongoing decisions about treatment and quality of life. I felt that, by documenting some of my journey, my reflections would not only give me the impetus to instigate the changes I needed in my life to minimise the risk of recurrence but that they might help someone else going on a similar journey.

When I began reflecting on the past year, I realised that I had learnt so much and in a relatively short period of time about topics such as surgery and treatment options, choice of a treatment team, emotions, effects on family and friends, stress, carcinogens, diet, exercise, meditation, support groups and seminars etc. The list became endless it seemed and the chapter became a book in no time. Thus, my challenge in preparing the present chapter has not been what to say but rather how to briefly summarise my journey and synthesize the main issues I need to confront in order to implement the changes in my life required for me to beat the dreaded 'C' and for good!

When I looked back at my 60-odd years of life, the main

theme that emerged was manic activity. The title of my chapter sums up the major issue I needed to confront – how to become a human 'being' rather than a human 'doing'. Pre 'C' I was not only a 'human doing' but I also inflicted considerable stress on myself. I was always busy; always organising people and events; always standing up for my rights; and forever pushing the boundaries.

During my school years I was highly motivated and studied as much as I could, often with little sleep. My parents didn't like me studying so much - after all I was a mere female whose role in life was to become a good mother and housekeeper! So, I saved my lunch money and purchased a torchlight so I could study under the blankets when my parents thought I was sleeping. I still remember my first boyfriend of some 11 years frequently commenting that he had to take a trailer with us when we went to the beach because I needed to have my books with me. He referred to Lyn 'in' and Lyn 'out' and that Lyn preferred to be 'out' and doing things. I am still the same even with my grandson – I would much rather take him out somewhere walking or playing in a park than stay at home with him. I even find it difficult to sit still enough to watch a movie; I could never be accused of being sedentary!

My study didn't finish at school – I spent 14 more years studying at universities and managed to complete two first-class honours degrees and then two PhDs.

Sporting activities were no different with simultaneous competitions in marathon and ultra marathon running (over 100km non-stop), masters swimming, marathon walking and long distance triathlon races – to the point where I looked anorexic.

So, my major challenge since being diagnosed with breast cancer has been to try to slow down and focus on 'me' and what 'me' needs in my life in order to nourish and heal myself. To reach this point of realising and implementing my major goal has required continued reflection and continual adjustments with baby steps, being mindful of the fact that, while I can't change the wind, I can adjust my sails. I knew that I had to keep my mind and body occupied but I needed to find a way to do this with less stress.

As I reflected on my 'human doing' behaviour and discussed this with the many women I had met through my journey, I progressively noted that I wasn't on my own. Almost without exception, the women I had met with breast and other forms of cancer have been high-powered, intelligent and highly success-ful. Moreover, every one of them has pinpointed stress as being a major factor in their lives leading up to their diagnosis. In fact, at a recent seminar on breast cancer, Dr. Boyle, an eminent oncologist, asked the large audience of breast cancer survivors to put up their hand if they had realised that stress had led to their diagnosis. The response was overwhelming – and if I had more than two hands, I would have put all of them up!

Yes, I am strongly of the belief that my breast cancer was directly related to the great stress I had always had in my life and then to the excessive stress I had experienced with moving 11 times between 2004 and 2010 when I was finally diagnosed in June of that year. Initially, I thought that there was little research data (beyond anecdotal evidence) to support my con-tention. Logically I knew that, when our immune systems are down, those little blighter cancer cells are given licence to grow because our body is unable to keep them at bay. I asked my breast surgeon and oncologist about my contention but their technical explanation of why I had breast cancer was "sh-- hap-pens" – meaning that we currently have little research data to pinpoint any particular causal factor.

Recently, in search of ways to minimize recurrence, I attended the week retreat at 'Quest for life' with Petrea King in Bundanoon for people with cancer and other life-threatening illnesses. One of the speakers at this retreat was a young man who had melanoma and was told in 2008 that he had only a few weeks to live. Still alive and well in 2011, this young man, who had followed the teachings of Petrea King, had spent the previous years researching factors related to cancer and he had reviewed an extensive body of literature including meta-analyses that provided evidence of a significant relationship between stress and cancer. So, my hunch and all the anecdotal evidence was finally validated! Then, the challenge! While I knew, logically, that I couldn't change the past, what did matter was what I had learnt from the past and how I could ensure that I no longer made the same mistake of inflicting stress on my body.

The retreat with Petrea King was critical to my journey with breast cancer. While I knew that I needed to de-stress my life, I had not taken on board the intuitive knowledge I had. I needed to learn how to relax – a skill that I had managed to fight against all of my life. During the retreat, we practised yoga and meditation every day and we did a seminar on music and movement. We took time to literally smell the roses in the garden, to laugh, to sing and to be creative. We were even able to indulge in relaxing massages and insightful counselling sessions. This experience made me realise how I enjoyed these activities and also how I had missed them because I was always too busy with work or some other stressful activity.

Petrea also talked about convalescence – a valuable concept from a bygone era that has become a luxury through economic rationalism, with hospitals rushing to discharge us as soon as possible, even with drains in. Of course, when we are discharged, friends and family assume that we are well enough to resume our domestic and work duties and we even convince ourselves that we can "get back into it". We seem to forget that we have not only experienced a tremendous emotional jolt with the diagnosis and surgery leaving us deformed and stripped of our womanhood but also that we have suffered physical trauma with all of the tests and surgery.

With little or no convalescence, we are then thrust into

seemingly endless investigations and treatment which debilitates us. Do we stop? No, we push on and the treatment takes over our lives. We count down until the end of treatment, thinking how relieved we will be. But, no, instead we feel vulnerable and uncertain – while we are being treated it's as if our boat is tied up at the wharf and then, when treatment is finished, we feel that our boat has been cut loose from the dock and is drifting aimlessly. How will I know if the cancer is back? We cringe with each twinge – is it back? Our doctors tell us that we shouldn't have further tests done for several months. The wait seems endless.

To make matters worse, our friends and family assume that we are 'all better' and can get back to normal. In any event, often they are tired of hearing about our illness – just like if someone says: "How are you?" All they want to hear is that you are fine; they don't want to hear any bad news. I am reminded of my loving and well-meaning daughter who wanted to delete the phone numbers for the oncology day centre and radiation oncology from my mobile. I wouldn't let her, with a shudder – not only had I spent a large amount of time in these venues and thus I felt separation anxiety but also I feared that I may need to contact them again in the future. To others we may be better but to us, no matter what anyone says, the fear of 'C' returning looms constantly in our conscience. So, the search for ways to reduce recurrence continues.

I don't know how some people manage to cope without taking advantage of the cancer support groups now available. I have been attending a support group with Life Force Foundation for the past year or so since I first heard about it from another colleague who was receiving chemotherapy at the same time as me. During our weekly support group meetings, we have an opportunity to share our concerns and joys in a supportive and confidential environment and then we engage in guided meditation to help us cope with the many issues associated with a diagnosis of cancer. These meetings have provided me with an opportunity to connect with and share my deepest emotions and to appreciate that I am not on my own. Moreover, I have learnt that I can help myself by helping others because showing empathy boosts our immune system. It's a win-win situation! Our group has bonded so well that we meet privately in the homes of participants when the official meetings are in recess. I know that I need never to feel alone; not only have my new friends had similar experiences to me, but also I know that they will listen to my concerns and provide me with the support that I need.

Life Force Foundation also provides a program for the carers of cancer patients. People caring for someone who has cancer often experience physical, psychological and emotional stress and thus self-care is just as essential for them as it is for cancer patients. In order to maintain their own health and wellbeing, carers themselves need to be supported.

Each year, the Life Force Foundation takes a small group of cancer survivors on a retreat where we are provided with a nurturing experience that helps to achieve and maintain a feeling of wellbeing. Research has shown us that emotional and psychosocial wellbeing supports the immune system and maximises the body's natural healing potential.

These retreats are facilitated by qualified counsellors and knowledgeable meditation teacher and participants are able to engage in a variety of activities such as vision quest, creativity workshop, massage, yoga and meditation, as well as delicious food. Moreover, the retreats are designed to facilitate confidential and empathic sharing in an enjoyable and relaxing environment.

I went on one of the retreats last year and experienced a profound sense of wellbeing through connection with the beauty of nature while enjoying nutritious food and delightful company. In fact, I gained so much from this retreat with a sense of healing that I have decided to attend a retreat this year as well.

On my journey I have also learnt the value of acupuncture combined with massage, with weekly sessions lasting at least 90 minutes. This treatment was invaluable during chemotherapy resulting in the boosting of my white blood cells and minimisation of nausea. After the active oncological treatment, I have found that acupuncture has been an extremely valuable adjunct to the medication I have to take to block the production of oestrogen in my body. Moreover, for me, acupuncture has been forced relaxation – I get a 30-minute relaxing massage before the acupuncture – and, it's not possible to move with needles all over your body!

The value of acupuncture prompted a search for relaxation exercises and meditation. Through another cancer survivor I was introduced to Qigong (a form of Tai Chi) which involves exercises to stimulate energy flow through the body combined with meditation and mindfulness. I started with one class a week and found the benefits so great that I now do three classes a week. Yes, I have been satisfying my life-long need to be active while at the same time relaxing!

I joined the Qigong master this year on a study trip to China investigating the benefits of medical Qigong. This trip introduced me to the value of traditional Chinese medicine and I was examined using these traditional techniques. A rather long script was prepared for me to help me combat the cancer. However, while the ingredients were translated for me, my concern was that I did not want it to interfere with the Western medicines that I prefer to rely on more heavily. Therefore, I chose to follow up the Chinese herbs with a Chinese doctor in Sydney who practices both Chinese traditional methods and Western medical treatments to ensure there was no interaction between the two forms of treatment.

I maintained contact with the breast care nurses at both hospitals where I was treated. What a fantastic service they provided from support to adjusting with no breasts (after having had DD-E size breasts since around the age of 12 years) to general information and referrals to various services. Even after I was discharged I knew that I could phone or email these nurses with any questions or concerns I had. They recommended the Encore program (gentle exercise for breast cancer survivors to get the body moving again after surgery and to minimize the risk of lymphoedema) and dragon boat training. I joined both of these programs as soon as I could after my treatment and through these activities I have met some stimulating and knowledgeable women with whom I have shared notes regarding useful treatments and programs. The Encore group meets on a monthly basis for a healthy meal and non-stop catching up, while I now train regularly with the special dragon boat team for breast cancer survivors. Dragons Abreast is a large national organisation with a huge membership of highly motivated survivors and their supporters. These women have a strong bond and provide invaluable support for each other.

Through these groups I have followed up contacts with a naturopath and a doctor who specialise in complementary medicine. I am taking a range of supplements to help alleviate the side effects of the oestrogen blocker I will be taking for many years to come and also to boost my immune system. I have found out that exercise is valuable but that excessive exercise can be detrimental. One of the main side effects of excessive exercise is an increase in oxidation – intensive exercise basically uses up our antioxidant reserves or we literally start to rust faster on the inside. I now realise that, if our levels of nutrients are low, it's difficult to replenish the necessary antioxidants and so there is an increase in free radical damage inside the body leaving us vulnerable to illness. I am now taking a supplement from the juice of olives. Research on this supplement has shown that it is the most powerful polyphenol antioxidant discovered to date (polyphenols are also found in green tea, red wine, cacoa and berries).

I investigated exercise options and, again through one of my cancer galpals, I was introduced to the local seniors' centre which offers a range of different exercise classes designed to put smiles on the faces of senior women. One of the classes is run by an energetic 80–something woman who can outmanoeuvre any younger woman at the centre. We do light weights and dance routines and then I do a tap dancing class with her. I was a tap dancer in my very early years, and I feel like a teenager again during this class.

I had wanted to try Zumba for a while but thought it was too strenuous and just for 'younguns'. I then found 'Zumba Gold' through the seniors' centre which is designed specifically for seniors and realised that I enjoyed the exercise within dance routines. This activity put me in touch with other women with whom I have bonded and shared experiences. Most of all, these classes are fun!

My new contact networks have introduced me to several research projects investigating factors related to breast cancer and I signed up for two of them. One of the studies is investigating the relationship between osteoporosis and exercise and the other is focusing on lifestyle factors and their link with breast cancer. Through these studies, I am not only contributing to the research necessary to reduce recurrence in the community in general but I am also learning new skills.

So, my journey continues, day by day, with new lessons about 'me' and new findings about ways to reduce recurrence. I am less of a human doing and much more a human being and I have learnt that, while I can't change the wind, I can adjust my sails and I adjust them constantly. I have also learnt that life is not about waiting for the storm to pass; it's about dancing in the rain!

Kay's Story

Cancer is a vicious, stealthy, frightening, impoverishing, bitch/ bastard of a disease. The destruction of your life as it was hurts like hell. Cancer affects every aspect of everything for you, your family and friends. The ripple effect is shocking.

For us, the pain of treatment was accompanied by a significant financial deficit. We lost money — in earnings, gap payments, hospital charges (over and above private insurance), chemist bills, parking fees, and in so many other ways. My income at first diminished considerably, then became intermittent, ceasing during hospitalisations and recovery, and then ceased completely under the strain of the disease.

My cancer journey, had I but known it at the time, commenced in 1999. I had persistent left-sided abdominal pain. The very first test my GP sent me for, a urinary tract ultrasound, reported back that the left kidney was smaller than the right, but 'within normal limits'. Wrong! The kidney was shutting down due to a tumour blocking urine flow. Unfortunately this was not finally discovered until early 2001 when I had a dramatic urinary bleed and the diagnosis and treatment process started in earnest. I had struggled for eighteen months feeling ill with a diagnosis of irritable bowel syndrome. It has since become clear to me that the reading of scans and x-rays is more an art than a science, and that mistakes are common.

The diagnosis was a huge shock. Before I knew where I was surgery was underway. The result, initially, was apparently successful. The tumour was reported to have been contained within the urinary tract, with no obvious spread. I recovered slowly, feeling grateful that things were no worse. However, my employers were unconscionably harsh. I subsequently discovered that when they heard the diagnosis they had tried to find a way to sack me. The atmosphere in the office after I returned was poisonous, so I found another position, which was part-time at a greatly reduced salary, in order to escape an untenable situation.

However, the dream recovery run was not to continue. By Christmas of 2001 it was determined that I actually had a lung secondary, and the question of treatment once again pushed us through a fresh round of consultations and tests. The lung secondary was treated with thermal ablation (heat-generating probes inserted directly into malignant tissue) in March 2002, and then a long round of chemotherapy ensued, lasting until November. Shortly after the thermal ablation I was diagnosed with a pulmonary emboli. I was admitted to emergency and then discharged on warfarin. When I had been home a fortnight my specialist rang. Having reviewed the scans again, he decided I hadn't had a pulmonary emboli at all. This business of radiological inexactitude has continued throughout treatment, with every fresh CT finding or losing something different.

Next came chemotherapy. This was commenced in March 2002, and lasted right through to November. My new boss, a cancer survivor himself, was kind and encouraging, and without his support I would at that stage have stopped working. So I continued part-time, and we quickly learned to have a stand-in on fixed days post-chemo.

The chemotherapy nurses in St. George Public were magnificent. They were purposeful, efficient, friendly, compassionate, and worked hard in appalling physical surroundings. At the time I was there the chemo room was equipped with dud chairs, curtains that didn't match, a TV that didn't work and a water-stained ceiling. It was badly designed as well, with the work desk in the worst possible position, so that every time a drip beeped (and that is nearly all the time) they had to hunt it down from the far corner of the room. I actually wrote to a home renovation TV program, in the hope that they would re-decorate for this great team, but no luck. For my own part, and recognising the team effort of the nurses, I always tried to accept the treatment as beneficial and kept positive, in the belief that in some way this may help them in a very challenging job.

During this stage, I began to attend a weekly group called Life Force. They are there to provide emotional support for people with cancer. I attended my first meeting in a state of great confusion and apprehension, with no thought of anything other than how bad I felt. After a while, I was able to look at things a bit more clearly, and feel that I was not so alone. Often the last thing you want to do is burden your family with any additional load, and at the Life Force meetings, I was able to talk without any fear of hurting someone I love. No one preaches or tells you how you should be feeling or what you should be doing or which other doctor you should be visiting or which other avenue you should pursue. Whatever state you are in and whatever you are saying or doing, it's acceptable and okay. After a while, I was able to see outside of myself, and discover real friendship with people travelling the same path as myself.

Post–treatment has its challenges. Due to the experimental nature of my treatment – radio frequency ablation – follow up CTs were frequent. So in a sense I was never able to shed the illness. There was always another appointment, another test, more questions answered – largely because the cancer was expected to re-appear. It is difficult to move on with life when you are pulled back all the time.

In October 2005, a repeat scan showed peritoneal regrowth. There followed more tests, the worst of which nearly gave me a heart attack. The registrar taking a biopsy sample declined to anaesthetise, even though I had fasted and prepared for anaesthesia. He removed several samples of tumour with no attempt at analgesia. The pain was so severe, that for the first and only time, I made a complaint to the hospital, telling them that the man was unfit to work on live patients. They apologised and offered to retrain him. I hope they did!

Subsequent major surgery showed a completely new cancer had suddenly developed. I went from worrying about a recurrence of transitional cell carcinoma, to having peritoneal cancer. Chemotherapy was commenced only a week after the operation, in November 2005, and it continued till October 2006. Once again, the chemo nurses in St. George Public were brilliant. But the TV still didn't work, the curtains still didn't match (strange that I find this so very irritating), the ceiling was still stained, the room is still a logistical nightmare, the chairs were even more uncomfortable, and those nurses were busier than ever.

The only break during treatment was when my PICC line got infected, and I was an in-patient for a fortnight with septicaemia. During this admission, I found myself in a mixed cancer ward, directly opposite a poor man who was only days from death. The experience was obviously depressing because I wasn't just worrying about being on intravenous antibiotics and having a life threatening infection. His family had to visit and grieve in a four-bed ward until a single room finally became available for him, and I was both confronted and challenged by watching the potential end of my own illness, and the way it would impact the people I love the most.

Chemo the second time round has not been successful. While the tumour markers fell, meaning the tumours had declined in activity, at no point did the drugs reduce the size of the cancer. The bastard is still there, and now I am about to re-commence treatment, this time starting with chemo and then more surgery. I feel like I have lost a year. And at 60, years are precious.

The worst aspect of this is the constant effect on the people you love the most. You cannot protect them. You cannot shield them. You have to let them in, knowing that they need full information, even when it is hurting all of us. Different family members react differently. Some take on the pain so much they themselves become seriously affected with depression. Some maintain perspective and offer frequent support. Some are so far in denial that when you ask for help they say, "I'm busy, but no worries, you're going to be just fine!" My immediate circle of friends has been fantastic, sticking there through thick and thin. The threat of yet more surgery has pushed me into unemployment. And next year, in addition to treatment, we have to face the fact that reduction in income equals a move from our small home into something cheaper. It is hard sometimes to find the positives. But that is the only way to stay sane.

Never give up.

Angel's Story

Angel Ioannou

At first I thought the small lump in my neck was a result of my lymph glands swelling up from a minor infection. After it remained for several weeks my GP recommended a visit to my specialist.

I had a bit of a history over twenty years before with 'lumps and bumps' that weren't malignant. However, the tests I had in November 2000 showed otherwise. Once again I had to start dealing with the whole thing. Why me? Will I live? What of my wife and family? How do I tell my mum? How do I just explain to people I have cancer? What do I do? What type of treatment should I have? Maybe they're wrong? Yes, I should get a second opinion. I'll take better care of myself.

I initially felt overwhelmed by the amount of information and number of decisions I needed to make. After diagnosis, I started to learn a new vocabulary including 'non-Hodgkin's lymphoma', the names of the chemicals used in chemotherapy and their effects, treatments, 'autologous transfusions' (using my own blood), stem cells and more.

As I talked to people, watched TV or walked down the street I thought to myself, *I've got cancer and you haven't*. It wasn't that I was angry at others; it was just that I felt different and a bit isolated. It wasn't that loved ones or people were the cause, it was just how I felt.

At times it seemed the diagnosis via tests and the surgery were much more painful and scary than the lump in my neck. But it was all part of it, as were the endless blood tests and needles for pushing or pulling chemicals and blood samples.

In January 2001, I started a regime of chemotherapy that involved a visit one day a month to the hospital where I received a chemical cocktail via intravenous drip for around five hours over a period of five months.

I felt okay and the anti-nausea drugs worked well for me. I was able to continue working and this provided a great distraction for me. My job at that time was in a consultative IT role across Asia Pacific and I was able to travel managing this schedule with the needs of the treatment.

Yes, I was feeling okay. After the second treatment I left to present at a conference in China and then travelled to my company regional sales conference in Bangkok. The party night had a 1950s theme and my roommate coloured his hair jet black and I did the same with the remainder of the dye. It was a fun night but I was tired and retired early and as the night was hot, I had a shower to cool down and wash my hair. As I was washing I became aware that my hair was falling out. That was a low point; my doctor had told me it would happen but I had no idea of how or when. It was a real stark reminder of living with cancer. In some ways I think I was in a state of denial. I was thinking I'm getting treatment, I'll be alright. But here was physical proof that everything was not alright.

The next day I flew home as scheduled and then decided it was time to deal with my hair and try dealing with my head. Having my hair cut right off was the easy part; dealing with my head was harder.

When all this started I was already researching my options in regard to possible treatments and reading about other people's experiences on the internet. While some stuff that I read was informative, there was also an awful lot of crap on the web including, I think, false hope and bogus treatments.

The treatment continued for another three months until the chemotherapy program ended. Then it was time to take more tests, mainly blood tests and CAT scans. I was optimistic, I mean I'd had the treatment, I was in good hands; we knew what we were treating.

The CAT scan showed that far from halting the growth, the reverse had occurred. The growth had increased and spread further with new tumours in my lungs and liver.

My wife and I were shattered. My specialist recommended operations to get samples from my lungs and liver to determine if they were the same or different. At this point I decided to stop working. I couldn't concentrate on anything. I was unsure of myself and feeling very low and this rubbed off on my wife. This period was my lowest point. I'm the type of person who gathers information, decides on an action and then tries to carry it out. I had two operations in one month and the make-up of my cancer was proving elusive, which made it hard to determine the best approach and treatment.

My doctor advised another three rounds of chemotherapy treatment, each of a much stronger and longer dosage, which would require hospitalisation over a ten week period.

The treatments occurred and I tried to just take it day by day. I read a lot and listened to music which was all to help distract my mind from the endless cycle of, 'what's next, will it work, will I live?'

Sleeping at night was getting hard as my mind would race through all manner of thoughts. My brain just ran amok at times.

During and after all this treatment I tried to make sense of everything, find meaning, peace and direction but it was a real struggle. Towards the end of my stay in hospital, I watched the Tampa affair on the news and then most of the collapse of the World Trade Centre. I felt very strange at the end of the treatment. It's hard to describe but I imagine it's similar to people who have had a very tough period and suddenly part of it ends but it doesn't really.

After the chemotherapy I was put on a trial of a new drug that required a morning visit (once a week over four weeks) to the clinic where the drug was intravenously fed into my body over three hours.

After this I had CAT and PET scans. The results were very, very good. The growths had either gone or were tremendously reduced. That was a great day. My eyes are welling up just writing that sentence. Although I was ecstatic and greatly relieved, I still had an emotional restlessness that I needed to deal with.

All the staff at the hospital, the doctors, nurses and support staff were fantastic and supportive, to a degree. It was out of their scope and time to help me deal with my ongoing emotional feelings. I thought of joining some type of support group and the social worker at the hospital gave me the Life Force Cancer Foundation phone number.

From the first call I was confident that this group could provide the right type of support. I joined the weekly Annandale Group that was just starting up a new term. The spirit of the group was facilitated by a counsellor who provided a trusting environment to let out our feelings and share our emotional experiences. Each week at the end of the session we all joined in meditation with the other facilitator, to help ease our minds after the sharing session. I looked forward to my weekly session with the others and slowly started to feel more relaxed with my cancer experience.

It has taken me more than four weeks to write this short account of my experience and it has been almost six years since I finished my treatment. It is still not easy to relive the experience but one of the most important decisions to help myself was to join one of the Life Force support groups. Even though it is also about six years ago, the help and support I received there continues on in my life today.

A New Journey Begins

Brent Couper

It was the end of 2005. We were sailing smoothly, Joy and I. Approaching 60 years of age, we could look back and feel very lucky. Good health, interesting jobs, great families and us, together. We began to 'downsize', contemplate early retirement, or at least part-time volunteer work, and getting on with our 90-year life plans.

In 2006, we started looking for that magic apartment, a safe harbour for our next decade. We put our dear home of 15 happy years on the market, found an ideal spot, sold up, and packed for the move.

Joy saw our doctor. "Not to worry," she said, "just a minor stomach upset." But the tests said otherwise. Stage four bowel cancer. "Without treatment you may have only six months to live." Bugger!

Was it a shock to discover cancer? Well yes, but not as much as I had thought. The tests, the research, the chats had warmed us up to the possibility. The real shock for me was the part about six months — she could be gone by Christmas! Now cancer was reality.

What next?

There's so much to learn and in a 'foreign' language — the medico language, big words and new concepts. So many decisions: which doctor, which treatment, which drugs, when, for how long, where? The list goes on.

How do we tell our families, our friends, our work colleagues? What do we say? When? Will our youngest grandkids understand? Probably not, so we decide not to try.

Joy had major surgery the week before we moved out of our home. Friends offered help and advice. Fellow patients shared their journeys and advice — reassuring, but overwhelming.

Joy tries new routines, an even better diet, more meditation, more regular exercise, as well as chemo cycles every two weeks. She sleeps, showers and works with her chemo drip attached. She smiles.

'Cancer' is such an emotional word, people try to be polite, but they are already sorry for you. Joy just wants to get on with life; unknowingly they 'coffinise' her. They talk as if the end is inevitable and near.

And then, during this, my Dad dies, suddenly. I put him to rest, with tears. I have his ashes in my hands and Joy is in hospital. And I think, how long before I have to put Joy to rest? Is it six months? Tears interrupt my answer. But I can't stop myself from mentally planning a funeral, thinking of parting words, just as I'd done for Dad.

The sailing is really rough now. The boat of my life, of our lives, feels out of control. Lots of tears, still.

Joy attends a Life Force Patients' Group and I attend a Life Force Carers' Group. We meet others in the same boat. It's nice to be able to talk, to listen, and to give and receive.

As a carer, I am learning a new language and a new role. I learn the important difference between helping, fixing and serving — when you help, you see life as weak; when you fix, you see life as broken; when you serve, you see life as whole. I learn the difference between being helpful (responding to what Joy needs) and being the helper (what I think needs to be done). I find these distinctions useful as caring, really caring, adds a new dimension to loving.

I hear "diagnosis is an opinion, not a prediction". I learn to question the statistics, which is useful and comforting, especially when the statistics of cancer can be so confronting.

My expectations about life are changing, though I realise that

I didn't think of them much BC (before cancer). Before, I felt that Joy might out live me as I'm male and older. Now I'm not so sure.

We both attend a workshop on 'Embracing Life While Facing Death'. We meet fellow voyagers, patients and carers, and reflect together for two days. It was a very gentle yet powerful experience for me, so early in our new way of life. We are encouraged to think of our situation as a journey we travel, not as a battle that we win or lose.

Complementing this, we hear that, "Death is certain, time of death is uncertain". In a strange way I'm comforted by this. Serendipity lessens the certainty of anything. We discuss how to balance hope and realism, we need both. Yet if we are too hopeful we are out of touch; if we are too realistic, we risk being morbid and giving up. The phrase, "Hope for the best, plan for the worst", works well for us.

By late 2006 life has settled down pretty well. We are in that new apartment, and it is magic. It will do very nicely for the next ten years. Will there be ten?

There's a rhythm where the cancer treatment becomes part of our life. There are fewer surprises, diaries settle down somewhat, we know what to expect, sort of.

The chemo cycles which started at every two weeks, now become three weeks and then four as the chemo takes its toll. Joy's body needs more rest. She still smiles. A resilient gentleness radiates. I sometimes marvel at how she does it.

Our wills and finances, which needed changing, are almost sorted out —we can relax on that front.

We finally decide to make that trip in May next year — a conference in China and holidays in Japan with friends. Up until now we weren't sure that we could make it — would Joy's health be good enough, would she even be here?

Christmas 2006, is a very important time. Joy asked the whole family to come to Christmas at our new home. They came from everywhere and we had a great day, including the concert put on by the grandkids. Left unsaid was the question, "Is this the last Christmas with Joy?" It gave the day a special meaning.

It was a celebration too, the six months had passed and Joy was here and doing really well. Yet there was also sadness for me. It was the first Christmas where, despite all Joy's family being there, I was alone, all my immediate family gone.

Then in early 2007, after eight months of treatment, we receive good news, very good news — Joy can take a break from chemo. Our trusted oncologist feels the results have been great so far, good enough to stop for a while and see what happens — partial remission.

We take that holiday, it was great. Living 'normally' is wonderful, as you can easily forget what it is like.

I see my skin specialist, "Not to worry," she says, "just a rash". I see a physiotherapist about pain in my right hip, "Not to worry," she says, "just a little arthritis".

The rash gets worse and the hip is still painful. Blood tests confirm Stage four non-Hodgkin lymphoma. Bugger! Again! I joke, "I'll have what she's having!" But I don't really mean it. It feels like we're part of a Monty Python skit!

This was not meant to happen. I was meant to be strong and able to care for Joy. Now things are topsy-turvy. "Death is certain, time of death is uncertain," I muse, again.

What next? There's so much to learn and so many decisions — new hospital, new staff. Again how do we tell others? Friends are devastated by our 'double act' and offer to help. Fellow patients share. New routines and chemo cycles every three weeks.

In a perverse way, I'm glad Dad has gone. He lost his daughter to cancer when she was 40 years old. I wouldn't want him seeing his son also experiencing cancer.

Now Joy is my carer. She explains that for her being a carer is much worse than being a patient. Seeing your loved one suffer is worse than worrying about your own health. Her words stay with me, "When you were diagnosed it was a kick in the guts. I felt fear. I felt helpless. With me being sick I may not be able to look after you". With hindsight I didn't realise the full extent of Joy's despair. I hope I do now.

Joy is also my coach and because she has led the way my journey is much easier. Now I attend the Patients Group. I've 'crossed over', as they say. Still, I can now appreciate both sides of the fence.

The second time around the sailing is not as rough. We've been on this type of voyage before. Together we've experienced the waves and cross currents, and learned how to navigate them better.

Joy's one last stubborn tumour has begun to grow and she now needs more chemo. Realism bumps into hope for a while. Both of us are attending different hospitals at different times, with different routines and different doctors.

We accept the many changes in treatment days and dates. Good diary management is essential. It seems we now take turns at being the carer, depending on who's had treatment recently. We are working together, each looking out for the other, anticipating each others' moods and needs. There is a strange new dimension to the very loving and respectful bond between us.

So here we are. The water is rougher than we imagined 18 months ago and the wind less predictable. The will is still strong, but the sailors are less certain. The goal is the same, but the journey is different now. A new journey has begun.

A New Language

Giulia Priante

There is only me, my husband and our three children here in Australia. We moved from Italy in July 1991. Then in 2000, when my youngest child was only seven years old I was diagnosed with breast cancer.

I had a mastectomy, then chemotherapy which made me very sick. I was scared I was going to die. I felt completely alone and was terrified.

I tried to find some support through various Italian associations, to see if I could talk to anyone else going through a similar experience, but I couldn't find anything to help me. Trying to come to terms with what had happened without any help from outside my family made me feel impotent and withdrawn. My worst agony and torment was at night when I couldn't sleep. I was distraught, thinking that I might die. My family did what they could, they tried their best, but my fears were too big for them to be able to help.

When chemotherapy finished I was very depressed, nervous and anxious. No one I talked to wanted to hear about this. I still wasn't sleeping and was still scared I would die. Then a friend called Anouche, who I met at a meditation centre, told me about a support group run by the Life Force Cancer Foundation. I will always remember Anouche because without her telling me about Life Force, I never would have started on my road to healing. I also met Lucia, another Italian lady who also went to Life Force, and we have become good friends.

I contacted the people in charge straight away and started going to the support group in Annandale. When I started there

I was very worried that people wouldn't understand me because my English isn't very good. But with Jane and Caro and the other group members I felt comfortable and accepted even when I knew it was sometimes hard for them to understand me. I never felt any judgment. I found a group of wonderful people and I realised that even though our first languages were different, we all spoke 'cancer'.

Right from the first meeting I felt reassured. I remember after that first night I finally managed to sleep right through the night after many, many sleepless nights. I heard that quite a lot of the other people had problems sleeping too. It was extremely important to me, listening to the others' experiences, realising that they were similar to mine. I felt much less alone and slowly noticed that I was changing the way I dealt with cancer and with myself. I began feeling stronger and stronger; my fears began to diminish and whenever I went home after a support group meeting I felt full of positive energy. Even my family noticed these changes in me and this led to being able to talk about my problems in a much more relaxed way. I even found myself dealing with them in a less dramatic way. For an Italian being less dramatic is a huge change!

In the group I learned about creative visualisation and I still use this because I find it very useful. I have never forgotten my first meeting and the beautiful garden that Caro took us to in our minds. This stuff is now part of my life and even if I don't use it every day I know where to go when I need to find a peaceful place. I believe in this very much because it works for me. I went to my support group for a year and even now I still go back every now and then because I don't want to lose the sense of connection and friendships I made there.

Since I started with Life Force my personal life has changed a lot. I never knew anything about counselling before because Italians don't usually have counselling. Counselling in Italy only started to develop in 1990. I found the type of counselling offered at the Life Force groups very gentle and compassionate because it is person-centred. I'm now in my fifth year of a diploma course, learning this same type of counselling. I've learned to stay with my feelings when it seems they need exploring whereas before I would have suppressed them or displaced them. Maybe this is one reason why I got cancer. I had a very difficult childhood that affected my whole life as an adult in my role as a wife and mother. I feel I'm a different person now and I wouldn't have become that person if I hadn't found Life Force.

I have also attended many Life Force retreats. The thing that attracted me about the retreat is that we were there just for ourselves and we were free to just feel whatever came up. In this way you feel more yourself because you don't have to hide anything or pretend to be a way you think others expect you to be. You don't have to 'disappear' within yourself. Sometimes I used to wonder where I had gone.

One of my favourite activities at the retreats is an American Indian ritual called a 'Vision Quest'. Every time I have done this I have learned something new about myself. I haven't been able to go to a retreat for a couple of years but I would love to be able to go to at least one every year because I feel good for up to a year after each one.

I will never forget the support I got from Life Force and it has changed my life in a very positive way. I have learned to overcome my fears and anxieties. It is now much easier for me to cope with issues concerning the relationship with my partner, the fear of death and problems which could come up if my cancer comes back. I have gained a sense of self. I've built new ties with people and I have more confidence in myself. I am a much happier person. I think about the future with more serenity, whatever happens. I live life appreciating all that is given to me. I have found myself and am living a better life than I ever had before.

When I graduate with my counselling diploma I hope that I can provide similar support to other people, especially in the Italian community. I would like to run an Italian-speaking support group the same as the Life Force group.

I will always be grateful to Life Force, especially Jane and Caro, but also all the other people I've met who shared my journey with me.

Note: Giulia now has her Diploma in Counselling and is available to talk to anyone in the Italian Community who is dealing with cancer.

Who am I? Big question

**Jane Gillespie, Counsellor and
Support Group Facilitator**

Where do I start, back to the beginning, back to the past.
Second child, second daughter, Roger I'm not. It's okay though, I'm
cherished; dressed like a doll in hand-fashioned clothes made by Mum.
Who am I? Big question.
Grow up shy, often lonely. Can't compete with big sister. To find an
identity, marry at twenty — better grab him or my chance might
have passed.
Can't conceive, feel a failure.
Then light of my life, my beautiful son, comes into my world by way
of adoption.
Loved daughter then follows and seven years on
a miracle happens. My own baby is born.
Failure again, my child is not perfect. No acknowledgment of grief,
just accept and move on.
Who am I? Big question.
Had to be the best mother, despite my pain.
Years of hard work, one thing is now plain — can't be all to others.
Not there for myself, I pay a high price.
Husband leaves for another. I gain some insight.
Who am I? Big question.
Next challenge is cancer and mad
as it seems, find the key to the
door at last. I push the door open — goodbye to the past.
Who am I? Good question.
Sometimes I am joyous and sometimes I'm not,
courageous or fearful, ice cold or red hot.

I am bold, I am timid, I'm strong or I'm weak.
At times I am sassy at others I'm meek.
I might be grown-up, but sometimes feel small.
I can rage or accept, or not BE here at all.
I'm human and fallible,
sometimes good, sometimes bad,
I'm angel or monster, but accept all I am.
The main thing I've learnt, it's
okay to feel — I'm finally me
AND I'M FINALLY REAL.

Abandoning Control!

Jann Chambers

I am writing this on the fifth anniversary of my surgery for breast cancer. There have been plenty of times when I wondered if I would make it this far. Even at this point, which is auspicious in terms of the medical world's statistical way of thinking, I know how fragile we are. I do not take my life and future for granted, and after the process of the past five years, I can never go back to being who I was. I am content with this, but it didn't start that way five years ago.

I didn't imagine it would be me who got cancer. It was always older people or some swift tragedy that nobody on the outside got close to. I knew people had lived through it, but I didn't know how. I had never really understood the implications of a cancer diagnosis. I suppose I thought that it was the beginning of some kind of path towards an inevitable end. However, I knew this wasn't true for everyone. What would happen to me?

When I found I had a pretty risky breast cancer, it felt as though I held my breath for a couple of days. It was as though I had become someone else — a person who had cancer. I thought I should look different but I still looked the same. The physical changes would come later. There was fear, but it was more like a challenge to my whole identity. It made me realise just how much I had seen people with cancer as different from me. They were another category of person. I just wasn't in that group.

Well here I was, and there was no way out, it didn't matter how much I chose not to believe it. I just had to continue. The choices, I found out later, were much more about just how you went about living each day. There could be no more of the adolescent assumption that things would not change, that losses and death were a long way off, somewhere in the distant future.

Arrangements were made for surgery quite quickly. Going to hospital was quite a familiar thing to me, and no trauma. It was tough on my family but I seemed to be in a bubble where not much could touch me. This was some kind of shock I suppose. The bubble seemed to keep on protecting me and I eventually realised that I was still the same person and started breathing a little more normally.

The time of diagnosis and treatment is a very high time because of the emotional intensity, the attention you get, the busy round of appointments and momentous medical sessions where you get the news, good or bad. I never seemed to be alone, and that was good. Later, during treatment I spent long days alone at home, and that is when I did have some hard times.

The comfort I gained from the survivors, who assured me that I would be all right, had a complex effect. Just look at them! They were fine. I had an extremely ambivalent set of reactions to this. On one hand wanting to take the comfort offered, and on the other knowing that from now on, kidding myself that I had any certainty about the future was no longer possible. This I had to learn how to accept.

The most difficult times were at night, trying to sleep. One miraculous night, after a period of tense lying awake, I managed to roll on my side and relax a little, and at that moment a beautiful physical memory of being held safely when I was a baby came to me. There was no doubt that it was a comfort from my mother. I was not thinking or trying to make myself feel better at that moment. It just arrived. I don't think I could consciously recreate that if I wanted to. It was much more about letting go, abandoning control or the attempt to understand the moment rationally, and recognising and accepting the feeling for what it was.

A very important moment came, late at night, when fear seemed just about to suffocate me. Ironically it was from this deepest moment of despair that the most change in me was able to happen. In the darkness, in deep fear of annihilation, something shifted. I felt better, somehow not alone and in some way I knew that whatever the outcome would be, at that moment I was fine. I truly think that it was at this moment, I began to develop a larger picture of my place in the universe. I let go fears of annihilation because I truly experienced the sense of being a part of some enormous whole. I now put much less emphasis on my individuality. These feelings were backed up by my readings in Buddhism and by other experiences while mediating.

Even in the early days my feeling was that deep down I was going to survive this. There was a cautious voice that said I was being over confident and that anything could happen but there was no help in brooding on fearful thoughts. I made a conscious decision to push away negative, repetitive thoughts. There was no point in them. My argument to myself was that if I was to get well, I would have wasted my energy and time on maintaining lousy feelings. If not, I would have wasted my remaining time on feeling lousy. So I fought it. I would catch myself going over and over some fearful thing, worrying about a pain, or a bump. Then I would push the thought away, or plan something that I could do to check it out. Even when I knew that a certain pain was explainable in other terms but advancing cancer, I could still catch myself repeating the fearful litany.

I had a friend and neighbour who had had the same experience a year ahead of me. She was a great support and told me about Life Force. I didn't immediately start to go to meetings. I was reading a lot about health, complementary treatments and most importantly, spirituality. I also had and still have a wonderful family and a group of supportive friends who visited, took me places, found me books and generally loved me. My work mates were also excellent, and kept me up to date as much as I wanted to be. I had decided to take time off work, to reduce stress and to allow me to have space and time to follow up treatments, appointments, exercising and reading.

I wasn't sure I needed to go to a group. I had found a wonderful little gaggle of neighbours, mostly elderly Greek women, and Mario the Italian bloke, who were doing Tai Chi in the park near my house, led by our Vietnamese neighbour John and his wife Maria. We started each morning at 7am, and wobbled through a beautiful set of exercises. John was not able to speak English, nor was Maria and I still don't know their Vietnamese names. This did not matter. We communicated perfectly well. As things went on, and I lost my hair and wore hats they were not able to ask questions but I know they were concerned. That was a wonderful thing, and really helped me to start the day well. I was able to clear my mind, and feel balanced and cheerful. I now do Qigong, which is a form of exercise related to Chinese medicine and acupuncture.

I think I finally read something that indicated that support groups were of great benefit to participants. Also, it is not easy to share your experiences with close people. They worry, and you often do not tell it like it is for fear of them not being able to understand, or for fear of burdening them.

So one day I telephoned the Life Force number and asked about the meetings. My first group was in winter. I dressed up in my wig, which I wore for special occasions, and plenty of warm clothes. It was almost like a disguise, in case somebody got too close, or they mistook me for one of them.

I was apprehensive because I felt challenged about being with people who had a difficult prognosis. How do you deal with knowing that your life is to be cut short? How do you talk to people who are possibly in this situation?

I think that looking back now I have had these questions answered. I have learned from wonderful people how I might live with the prospect of death gracefully, calmly and even with a sense of humour.

The facilitators were warm and welcoming. The ground rules were good. Everyone who wanted to could speak, no one was to interrupt or give advice, and everyone was treated with respect. I had not done too much crying, not since the initial period after the diagnosis but I found myself letting go a whole flood of tears that night. It was a relief to be with people who did not need explanations, and did not feel apart from you as the one with the illness. We felt very human together and not like outsiders.

I met people who were grand survivors; women who had struggled through numerous recurrences of cancer, and a couple who would eventually die. The relationships were wonderful. Nobody demanded more than was able to be given, and what was given was open acceptance, the willingness to listen and the space to make your own decisions free of judgement or unasked for advice.

I attended the group for about a year, and also went on a country retreat. This experience truly brought a whole lot of things together for me, and also for other people on the weekend. There was a young woman who had had cancer quite a few years before, in her early twenties. She was coming to terms with the loss she felt of her young adult life. There were also stories remembering the importance of the retreats to some of the people who had since died. The atmosphere created was cleansing and healing.

I really experienced some big changes on that weekend. The first was an opening up of my neglected creativity. I painted, drew and dreamed.

Even more importantly, after many years, even before cancer I had struggled with religion and just what I believed in, and what implications for action it might have in my life. I often felt as though my spirituality was not good enough, that I should sacrifice more. This set up huge conflicts that I could not resolve. I did not want to preach or to leave my family but kept on fearing that this was what was required of me. I actually feel that this conflict that I pushed away from me for many years was a factor in my becoming ill.

As I have already described, I had begun to come to terms with this during some of my most difficult moments.

What happened on the retreat, during a wonderful ceremony called a vision quest was that I gained a realisation of how I could integrate spirituality into my life as I was leading it. I did not have to leave my family to become a proselytising disciple of any of the religions or even become a Buddhist nun in order to lead a balanced and spiritual life. This was a great relief. I'd already lost the hair once. That was enough.

So five years later, where am I?

I have a better understanding of myself and how and why I am in the world. I am at peace with my spiritual life, and continue to practise meditation, Qigong and to read, discuss, learn and grow.

I still struggle sometimes with maintaining an even keel. I can sometimes go down the pathways of fear and separation or self indulgence, but not for long.

I love my family and my friends, and spend a lot of time with them. I am trying to balance work, exercise, family life and friendships, fun, creativity, travel, community activities, and an openness to opportunities to be of use to other people. Sometimes I just like to lie about with a good book.

Jenny's Story

Jenny Santori

For all of us life can change in a matter of seconds.

We are all in constant denial about our mortality but there is one thing that is certain.

We are all going to die, we just don't know when and from what.

For me my life changed only a few weeks ago when my annual routine mammogram and ultrasound revealed what was described to me as a "friendly cancer; the best one to have!" Suddenly I am forced to confront my mortality, statistics of relapse and decide on the most effective treatment.

Now how does anybody feel after being told you have cancer? I was numb and in shock, terribly anxious and uncertain, and feeling like I had been handpicked —yes, handpicked — as most people don't have cancer. I felt like I was pulled out from my normal everyday life and somehow reinserted back into my world but feeling very different and alienated. A counselor at my support group who had also been diagnosed with breast cancer described her feeling of alienation as being separated by a plate glass window — you can see everything going on as normal, only you are somehow separated from it.

There was a lot of anger in the first few weeks, not so much now. I still look at my friends and strangers on the street and assume in my mind that they are all okay and that I am the only one who has had something terrible happen to me. My husband tries to assure me that everyone has to face some kind of misfortune in their live; an accident, a bad marriage, financial troubles or other health issues. It's just that at the moment

I think that cancer is the worst one of all and that I am still relatively young at 50 years old with so much more I want to do. The unfairness of it all! Having been the main caregiver to my ageing and dying parents and surviving my children's teenage years I deserve to be free to be me, but feel terribly deprived of being able to do so.

Your friends will try to make you feel better but sometimes, even though they mean well, they come out with such things as, "We could all be hit by a bus tomorrow". No, it is not the same, I'm sure the statistics are very different and we all know that being hit by a bus or car is not likely to happen. The fact of cancer is a definite.

After surgery you may be cancer free but you are no longer able to hide from the knowledge of mortality and death. Your friends are only trying to provide some comfort but some can't acknowledge what you are feeling and your experience is invalidated. You have to remember though that people, especially those closest to you don't really know what to say. They are coping with their own shock about hearing about you as well as questioning their own mortality. They are all well intentioned and don't want to hurt you. Some of my friends told me that my diagnosis has encouraged them to go for their mammograms or other tests earlier rather than later.

I didn't think that any cancer was friendly but had to console myself that it could have been much worse. A fine needle biopsy and core biopsy revealed 'DCIS', what I soon learnt is a 'ductal carcinoma in situ', because it is housed in a contained duct. It is indeed a much better cancer to have — if you are going to have one.

Pathology results after a lumpectomy confirmed the DCIS but also revealed an 'invasive cancer' — this did not sound friendly at all and I had visions of my body being completely taken over by an alien force over which I had no control. Every ache and pain was attributable to a cancer lurking anywhere in my body. Fortunately one of my close friends who is a doctor assured me that invasive only meant that it had invaded tissue outside the duct and did not necessarily mean that it had spread throughout my body.

I had to assure myself with the 'good news' in my pathology report after my lumpectomy which was a clear margin around the tumour and the fact that it was oestrogen dependant. This opened up another type of treatment, Tamoxifen, to bring on immediate menopause by starving my body, and hence the tumour, of oestrogen. Further good news followed after more surgery; the sentinel node was clear and further tissue taken out in a second operation still produced a clear margin. Every bit of good news has to be celebrated and I do count my blessings.

I am presently still waiting for more results. When my surgeon punched in my variables into a type of generic online calculator, up came a prognosis of 28per cent chance of relapse if I chose not to undertake any further treatment. With hormone therapy that made it a little better. Chemo improved the numbers even more.

All of a sudden I am a statistic, a cancer sufferer — where is the person I was? How could I now be part of a whole group of other people I did not know anything about? However, a trip to my oncologist was much more encouraging, with an opinion that I was at low risk and therefore not a candidate for chemo. He did suggest if I could afford it, that my tumour could be sent to the US for a much more detailed analysis of my type of tumour. It would be put into a database that more accurately reflected my tumour type and therefore come up with a much better directed prognosis and recommendation for treatment would be made easier. It cost a lot of money but knowing the additional information will give me much more peace of mind and help me decide whether I need chemo.

The waiting is excruciating; you are in a limbo land where you find it hard to focus and make arrangements too far into the future. I am told that this is the worst time as you do feel very passive and the uncertainty for me is very worrying. I am finding it a little easier now and am coping better with just trying to be normal and do all those normal things that I previously took for granted as so easy to do like shopping, cooking, working, being with friends and family, socialising, watching movies.

I am doing my best to cope with my diagnosis, operations, procedures and decision for treatment by reaching out for whatever support I can muster to give me strength at this time. I have met some people who soldier on bravely, who are less inclined to share with others; but who ultimately pay the price later. The Cancer Council was my first port of call. They have been warm, friendly and very reassuring. Just having a warm and compassionate voice at the other end of the line is so reassuring when you are feeling low or desperate. They also sent me literature on my type of cancer including treatments, food, complementary therapies and a whole heap more.

I tried not to read too much or go to too many websites as I believe a little information out of context can be very dangerous. Especially with my runaway imagination and internal negative chatter which thrives on any bit of information, magnifying it, exaggerating it and then believing in it. I also got information about support groups in my area as I desperately wanted to connect to others who are going through similar experiences. I wanted to connect because I felt so disconnected to my normal life — somehow I just didn't fit in as smoothly as I always had. Even though my husband, children and friends have been very supportive and caring I still yearned for a connection to a new type of normality; a normality where other people from all walks of life, all ages, also got cancer and were trying to 'fit into' their old lives and adjust and cope with their new lives. Even when you are 'cured' of the cancer (the cancer is in remission and you finish your treatment), you still need others who really understand that you have become a different person to who you were and the challenges of coping with life post treatment.

I have been going to my support group every Monday for the last three weeks. I feel that each time I go the connection between us is stronger. Last week we finished a few minutes early and instead of everyone rushing off to their 'normal' lives, we just all sat there experiencing the connectedness of a new normality to which we are all trying to adjust.

I am also trying all sorts of other support networks to help me cope with such a high state of uncertainty. An acquaintance of mine who had breast cancer the year before recommended an acupuncturist who had helped her with her anxiety, stress and nausea post-chemo. Having never gone before I was interested to try anything that gave me the feeling of more control over my life and at the same time help with my own anxiety. It has helped me relax and lift a huge load from my shoulders and chest — a lot of emotion I had been carrying since my parents' deaths a few years ago and the anxiety I am feeling about the cancer. A needle in the middle of my face, between my eyes, helped with my runaway negative internal chatter responsible for a lot of my worrying thoughts that simply carry me away to places I would rather not go. Last visit I felt a little heavy in the chest and was coughing a little — a needle placed in my back designed for my lungs also helped to clear this.

My breast care nurse was referred to me by my surgeon. She is a wonderful resource and source of comfort. She rings me every now and then, mostly after procedures and test results just to see how I am traveling and to offer advice along the away. It is also comforting to seek out other people who have gone through similar experiences. It helps to talk to someone who has finished treatment and is getting on with their everyday lives. It provides a glimpse of the light at the end of my tunnel and I am inspired by their faith and positive attitudes.

By trying all these avenues of support beyond family and

friends I am able to be proactive and feel more constructive and positive in my treatment. I still struggle to try and understand why or how this has happened to me. Was I too stressed? As the primary caregiver of my parents, did my perfectionist personality and sometimes negative attitude contribute to my cancer? I am a vegetarian, exercise often and don't drink or smoke. Could I have done anything differently to avoid this? If stress did contribute to my cancer, then why don't all stressed people get cancer? I think the best approach was beautifully explained to me by a work colleague. She explained that cancer is egalitarian and non-discriminatory and that shit just happens for no reason at all. Not to say that I shouldn't work on my stress levels and that I shouldn't start to view the world in a more positive and hopeful light.

One thing for sure is that the stuff at work or home I used to get stressed about does not upset me nearly as much. Having cancer is a very sobering experience that instantly puts everything else into perspective.

Whilst I was terribly angry at the world and God after my diagnosis, I no longer blame God for any of this. Random events just happen and God's role, I believe, is not to micromanage our lives. I do believe, however that He can give us strength and help us find direction in our lives. I do believe that He has given me a helping hand to help me deal with this. Random meetings with key people who have given me advice and the opportunity to use an office at work have helped me cope. For years I have worked in an open plan environment where it is hard to focus at the best of times. Offices are like hens' teeth at work but somehow the opportunity presented itself at a time when I needed it most. The day I was offered an office happened to be the day I went in for my mammogram!

I hope my story can help others cope in some way with their diagnosis and adjustment to their 'new normality'.

Destiny? Schmestiny!

Lynne Davis

My mother was diagnosed with breast cancer in 1971 at the age of 47. She underwent a radical mastectomy, hysterectomy, chemotherapy and radiation treatment. The effect on her life was severe but she survived the experience. However, when her cancer recurred 13 years later I think she felt unequal to the struggle and this time she did not survive.

Since her first diagnosis, I had always felt that in some way breast cancer was my destiny. From that time on, although young, I had annual mammograms and breast examinations. Cancer, when it came, stole a march on me. I had an emergency appendectomy following a ruptured appendix in 2002. When I attended for my post-operative appointment ten days later I was told that a carcinoma had been discovered in my appendix during routine pathology testing. I couldn't believe it. Here it was at last — my destiny — but looking quite different from what I had imagined. I have a very clear recollection of that moment in the surgeon's rooms, the icy rush of fear, the sensation of a darkening world, and the feeling that this was a movie which I had projected many times onto a screen in my mind.

It was a curious situation, really. My cancer was gone before I even knew it was there, but then I faced the prospect of major surgery and chemotherapy — not to remove the cancer but as a kind of insurance policy in case cancer cells had escaped with the rupture of my appendix. And so began a nightmare time of pain, extreme anxiety and fear. Not so much fear of death as of suffering, with which I was all too familiar following the deaths from cancer of my mother and my best friend some years earlier.

I won't expound on the physical experiences of surgery and chemotherapy here. The surgery was major. I believe abdominal surgery of this kind is amongst the most intrusive and painful. My chemotherapy, on the other hand, was among the less 'aggressive' kinds — that is, my hair did not fall out and I seldom vomited. All things are relative, including suffering. But regular ingestion of highly toxic substances over a period of half a year, for whatever reason, is scarcely compatible with normal life. Nine months after the initial diagnosis, when my course of chemotherapy ended, I was 30 kilos lighter, grey in both appearance and disposition, and too weak even to make myself a meal.

This was all very traumatic and I hope never to repeat these experiences. But they were the tip of the iceberg; the real trauma was much less evident. Within hours of being informed of my diagnosis (with no prognosis) I was shaking uncontrollably. Shaking which went on and on, without respite. I couldn't think of anything else for many months, and for a long time I measured my recovery in terms of the intervals between thinking about cancer. For me, I believe that the psychological suffering was greater by far than the physical suffering. And this is hardly surprising. What greater existential challenge is there than the knowledge, lived with every minute for months on end that one's body may or may not contain a time bomb?

The astonishing thing is that this greater suffering is so little acknowledged. On one of my first visits to the surgeon I mentioned my extreme anxiety. He was a sympathetic man, not insensitive to psychological pain but unable to deal with it himself. He prescribed sedatives and gave me the name of a hospital-based psychologist who worked with cancer patients. I saw this psychologist from time to time during the period of my surgery and post-operative recovery, and he referred me on to a psychiatrist who specialised in treating depression in people with chronic conditions. I found the consultations with each of these people therapeutic in an 'emergency' sense, but didn't feel they provided me with any profoundly different perspective on what was happening in my life, nor on the grand themes of life, death, suffering and meaning. Nonetheless, going to see them had an importance beyond the immediate life raft they offered me; they were a part of the process of me defining what my real needs were.

After I had recovered from the surgery and embarked on a course of chemotherapy, I began to give some thought to what had happened to me and how I had been affected by it. To me, and I believe those closest to me, one of the most alarming things which happened was the collapse of my self-confidence and sense of efficacy. I've always been a rather strong-minded and decisive person, but I became quite unable to make decisions or to act with any degree of independence. Even quite simple phone calls seemed to be beyond my capacity for a time. And, as it happened, during this time it became necessary for our family move from our home of more than 20 years. I barely participated in this move, either physically or psychologically.

Strangely, in writing this, I've omitted to mention a singular fact of some importance. For some years prior to my cancer diagnosis I had been losing my sight and the two experiences intersected in some very particular ways. To begin with, I had to confront the undoubted fact that one life trauma is no antidote against another. It's difficult to avoid feeling the injustice of a double whammy, but really such thinking is quite pointless. However, it's been my observation that the medical profession and its institutions are less able to accommodate disability than many other sectors of society and thus an intensive period of highly medicalised existence is more than usually frustrating and isolating for a person with a disability. To make matters worse, the loss of my sight seemed to be considerably exacerbated either by stress, anaesthesia, chemotherapy, or some combination of these. As a result, I felt that I was the passive recipient of 'treatment' — that is, things were being done to me, sometimes without explanation, because I had no role in making decisions about what was done, or about my priorities. I believe this general feeling was exaggerated by my blindness and the inability of the professionals giving the 'treatment' to imagine either what it might be like to be blind or the intersections between blindness and being a cancer patient.

A major issue for me was the unavailability of information in a format which I could read. Only about three per cent of all information available in print is produced in alternative formats such as Braille or audio, thus routinely depriving people like me of independent access to information about their world. I felt this most acutely as I began to experience the desire to take some control over what was happening in my life. Other people I met who were engaged in a similar search had information I could only dream about. Who knows whether my anxieties would have been allayed by greater access to information, or whether I would have found what I was looking for sooner? I do wish, though, that the choice had been available to me.

Largely relying on word of mouth, I explored a range of approaches to the situation in which I found myself. I contacted an ex-colleague who had survived a difficult cancer some years earlier and from her found out about the approach advocated by Ian Gawler and about the Life Force Cancer Foundation. Ian Gawler's books were widely read and discussed, but I was only able to obtain a copy of the first edition of his original book, *You Can Conquer Cancer.* This was a life changing event for me. The general approach outlined in the book, a combination of science, philosophy and spirituality, gave me a different paradigm for dealing with my life circumstances, and in particular with the grand themes which had seemed to be so neglected by the more traditional approach to cancer diagnosis and treatment. This way, I felt I had some choices about the way I lived my life — and death, if it came to that. Accompanied by my partner, I attended a ten-day residential course at the Gawler Foundation's centre in Victoria, and experienced something of a regeneration.

On my return from Victoria, I decided to follow up on one of my colleague's other recommendations and contacted the Life Force Cancer Foundation about their support groups for people living with cancer diagnoses. I joined a group which met weekly — a very small group, as it happened, because in my area of Sydney there has not been a strong response to this possibility. At the first meeting I attended, one of the other members of the group spoke about a practitioner of traditional Chinese medicine she had consulted and on further investigation of this approach I decided to incorporate the Chinese practice in my armoury of techniques.

I found that there were a number of similarities between the philosophy of the people running Life Force with the Gawler approach, in particular, an emphasis on meditative practice. The Life Force groups complemented the other paradigms to some extent, in that they paid attention to the emotional state of the person rather than merely focussing on 'beating' cancer. I attended the group meetings for about a year, as well as spending a couple of beautiful and therapeutic weekends in the NSW countryside with Life Force members, some of whom became quite intimate partners in the 'journey'.

It's almost five years now since my cancer diagnosis. Cancer is no longer a daily presence in my life, although I've been profoundly changed by the experience in a multitude of ways. Some of the people I met along the way remain presences in my life. They're not all alive today, but they affected my life in a real sense, and I believe that their approach to their own illness and death was enhanced by the philosophies we discovered together. I know my own priorities have changed as a result, and although at present it remains untested, I like to think that if faced with life's great challenges in the future, I will find a calmness and dignity which was absent in my encounter with cancer.

A Carer's Story

Meldi Arkinstall

Turning up to barbecues telling people you're reading a great book on death and dying may sound strange, but this is where I was at when my mother was dying.

I desperately needed support. I needed to be around people who understood what was happening and who were going through, or had been through, caring for a loved one as they died of cancer.

The books on death and dying by Elizabeth Kubler-Ross were enormously helpful, but they're books you only read when you really need to.

The only way I got through the 12 months of hell from when my mother was diagnosed with cancer to when she passed away was by attending weekly support group meetings held by the Life Force Cancer Foundation. The group I attended was for carers of cancer patients. In this group I found people who were also going through the rollercoaster of dealing with the fact that a loved one who had cancer was dying or might die.

Mum was diagnosed with ovarian cancer (stage III) in March 2004 and she died in March 2005. She had a big operation where much of the cancer was removed, but it had spread floridly throughout the abdominal area and the momentum made removing all of it impossible. Some nine months after diagnosis my Mum's cancer had spread to the liver. There was a huge tumour and it was inoperable.

I can still remember Mum's brave little face as she sat with me, her sister and the specialist and asked why they weren't going to operate. We sat and looked at the scan of her liver, which showed an enormous tumour taking up almost the whole organ. She was so brave. It was heartbreaking. She was dead three months later.

The rollercoaster of emotions experienced by a carer is difficult to describe. Of course I was upset that Mum was sick. But then I got angry — at her — for being sick. Then I got guilty about being angry, and I got depressed, and the cycle continued.

My parents divorced when I was seven and my father lives in Brisbane. My brother lives in Malaysia, so I was 'it' in Sydney. Looking after Mum was very demanding and through attending the groups I received advice on how to contact community nurses and other means of support. This was a lifesaver. Mum was not an easy patient; she was a fighter and was doggedly independent. She never (to my knowledge) accepted the fact she was dying, so we weren't able to discuss it with her, or ask her about things she would like to do or have done.

We couldn't tell her we'd miss her. But part of her knew. She'd sit there with her big brown eyes and say, "I love you to bits Mush (her nickname for me)". I knew what she meant. She was facing saying goodbye to me, my brother, and everyone she knew. It was difficult for us; it was unthinkable for her.

At the suggestion of the group, I made up a list of a few of my mother's very good friends who kept offering to help. I contacted each of them and told them a specific way in which they could help — it might be visiting Mum at home on a day I couldn't get there; simply calling her to say hi; or dropping in a meal.

My relationship with my mother was a difficult one. I had to work on drawing strong boundaries with her, and this became very difficult when she was sick. She would call me up and say she needed the electricity bill paid. When I got there she had a list of other things that needed doing and it took several hours. As difficult as it was, I told Mum she needed to get used to reaching out to other people besides me for help. This was very difficult for her as she was such a reclusive person and she was very proud. In the end I had to manipulate her a bit and tell her it was to help me, not her. Then she agreed to do it!

Relationships within my family changed a lot as Mum got sicker and the stress of the situation began to take its toll. She had two courses of chemotherapy and this made her very weak. At the end of the first course she was feeling a lot better and her specialist said she was in remission. He had done a blood test which showed a big reduction in the number of cancerous cells, but he hadn't done a scan. So we had a lovely Christmas celebrating. Then a few weeks later we found out there was actually a massive tumour.

My brother and I had a lot of tension during this time. We had always got on very well but I began to be angry about the fact that he lived overseas and that I was doing almost everything. This wasn't his fault but it certainly wasn't mine either.

This situation wasn't helped by the fact that my mother, who stayed in denial almost to the very end, told my brother by phone that everything was fine, and that she was getting better. He would then tell me I was being negative and making a big drama about everything. He planned a trip to the US for Christmas, based on what Mum was telling him.

Eventually, after support from the carers group, I made it clear to my brother it would be our mother's last Christmas and I told him he should come home as he might regret it in later life if he didn't. At first he was very angry and thought I was trying to make him feel guilty. But eventually he did come home and he was very, very glad he did. She died a few months later.

I was dealing with a very difficult boss during the year my mother was dying. She was picking me to shreds every day. My work went up and down as I was very depressed. Looking back, I have no idea how I got through it all without losing my job. I can honestly say I think attending the carers group was the main thing that helped me get through. Friends and family can only help so much, and then you need the trained help of professionals.

Thank you, thank you, thank you, thank you, thank you Life Force! I will never forget the help I received from everyone connected with the carers group.

The Pendulum

Nigel Bartlett

It seems like such a cliché, but I really do feel lucky to be alive. A miracle occurred for me when my cancer was discovered and removed before I even knew about it. Yet, despite my good fortune, I was left with powerful feelings of fear and bewilderment that at times seemed overwhelming, and that's where Life Force proved an unwavering pillar of support.

Having read a couple of books by Tour de France winner Lance Armstrong, who was 25 when cancer nearly killed him, I call August 26, 2005, my *carpe diem* day. That was when I went into hospital for an extremely minor piece of surgery, something I'd been putting off for years. But here I was, at 40, finally getting around to it.

The odd thing is that I didn't need to have the surgery. It was simply to correct something mildly embarrassing in an intimate part of my body. Twenty minutes under general anaesthetic, that's all it would take. I'd had a referral two years earlier, but hadn't followed it up, out of fear of the anaesthetic and procrastination. Even now, I wasn't sure I could afford the $500 I'd have to pay over and above what my health fund covered, and I'd been on the verge of cancelling the procedure because of that.

It turned out that it was the best $500 I've ever spent, and my earlier procrastination had produced wondrous dividends. If I'd had the procedure two years earlier, there would have been nothing else to find. On this day, however, when I came round from the general anaesthetic (an hour later in the end, rather than the planned 20 minutes), I sat waiting for the urology specialist to see me with my good friend Michele, who'd come to pick me up.

"He'll be with you shortly," said a nurse, handing me a sheet of photographs. Each one looked like pink moonscapes, a couple of them showing a series of ridges in a hand-shaped formation, others with what looked like a large crater in the middle. Michele and I peered at them. I don't know what was going through Michele's mind, but I just stared at them dully, my head still dazed and confused after the anaesthetic. I recall thinking the nurse had given them to the wrong person.

"You are an extremely lucky man," said the specialist, when he turned up to see me. "That," he said, tapping a picture of the hand-shaped ridges, "is a tumour. Bladder cancer. Although we won't know for sure until the results are back."

I stared at it blankly, too groggy for the effects to sink in. "And that," he continued, tapping one of the crater-like pictures, "is where I've cut it out with a laser and cauterised it."

"Okay," I replied.

"If we hadn't spotted it now, the first you'd have known about it would be blood in the urine — and by then it would've been the size of a golf ball."

Michele was more shocked than I was, until the next morning, once the anaesthetic had worn off. I didn't know what to believe. Was it really cancer? He'd said they'd have to wait for test results. Maybe I should wait until then to start worrying. Had they got rid of it all? Will I need treatment? Should I update my will? What do I tell people? *Do* I tell people?

Over the coming week, I emailed my parents in England, spoke to them on the phone a couple of times, and told a few close friends. My mind swung from one extreme to another. I'd swerve from all-consuming anxiety to telling myself I was making a fuss over nothing.

I went for the test results, accompanied by a nurse friend, Janet — on the very wise advice of my dad, who'd told me I needed another pair of ears as I wouldn't be able to take everything in. The specialist once again told me how lucky I'd been. Yes, it had been cancer. Yes, he was confident he'd removed it all. And yes, I'd have to have six-monthly check-ups, possibly for the rest of my life, because the chances of bladder cancer recurring are high.

Then he showed me a cross-sectional diagram of a bladder, with tumours of varying stages at different points around it, like the numbers on a clock. It proved graphically just how lucky I was.

"Yours was a stage-two transitional cell carcinoma." He pointed at one of the very early tumours, and then at one a bit further round. "When you get to stage four, that's the killer."

I was astounded at his language. Did he mean what I thought he meant? That just two stages further than mine (there were nine stages on the diagram), I would be a goner? For some reason (shock, most likely), I said nothing. I did ask some questions (and Janet asked several more), and the specialist once again congratulated me on my good fortune. I've since found out that getting to stage four means radiotherapy, chemotherapy, possible removal of the bladder, an ileostomy bag, and loss of erectile function. And yes, it means a high risk of death.

What was especially frightening for me was that, had my tumour not been discovered by chance, there's a strong risk it would have gone way beyond stage four. As the doctor had mentioned, the warning sign is blood in the urine, but I learnt later that many men ignore this, partly because the blood might be in such small quantities it's virtually unnoticeable, and partly because it may appear one day and not reappear the next, or the next — and partly because men generally don't like going to the doctor.

I rarely cry (I wished I'd cry more at times), but I did shed a few tears after seeing my specialist, with Janet sitting next to me on a sofa outside his consulting rooms. Sure, I was relieved, and grateful. Not just to the doctor, but to the universe, God, whatever it might be that had put me in his path at just the right time. But I was confused. I had cancer. No, I didn't have cancer. I'd *had* cancer, without even knowing about it, and now it had gone. Why was I feeling so shaky? What right did I have to feel shocked, upset? And what would I tell my parents?

I spent the next few weeks feeling at times elated, on top of the world, I'd never be afraid of anything, ever again. I'd ask someone out on a date without fear of rejection. I'd not fret about money, because money is just paper and metal. I'd jump out of planes, travel to South America on my own, I'd do anything, absolutely anything, because I'd had cancer and survived it, without having to go through any of the hideous treatments that others had to endure.

But just as quickly I'd snap into intense panic. What if it comes back? He said it was highly recurrent. What should I be eating, drinking, to make sure I stay as healthy as possible? Why haven't I had my skin checked for melanomas for the past five years? You idiot! What if I have some other form of cancer that I don't even know about? What's that ache in my arm? Did a bit of the tumour break away and metastasise, ending up in another part of my body? I had no idea whether these were irrational thoughts or not.

I made a flurry of appointments. I had a skin-cancer check-up (all fine, and I now make sure I go annually). I had myself investigated for bowel cancer (totally fine, but I'd seen some blood on the toilet paper a while back and I wasn't taking chances), I saw my GP about my arm and we considered having an MRI. And every doctor I came into contact with reassured me I wasn't over-reacting, it was worth taking all these things seriously, especially after my experience, and don't worry, we'll check them all out for you, make sure everything is fine. As for my arm, my specialist reassured me it was nothing to do with the cancer, and it was sorted out through visits to osteopaths and chiropractors.

I've realised through all this that I have fantastic friends, and one day one of them told me about Life Force, which she'd heard about while training to be a counsellor. I found the website, saw that meetings took place not far from me and phoned one of the numbers listed.

I really wasn't sure if I had any right to go to a cancer support group — after all, I no longer had cancer. But at the end of that phone call I felt confident enough to turn up at my first session in Annandale the following Thursday. What I found was a place where I could talk about things that I felt I had no right to talk about anywhere else — my confusion over what I 'should' be feeling, how to handle things when people didn't always 'get' what was going on for me, and the strange, unexpected thoughts that came into head from time to time.

While friends have been almost universally supportive, they have their own lives to live and don't always think to ask me how I'm going, and I've learnt that that's fair enough. Some of them didn't fully understand what had happened. One of them asked a while later, "So, was there a name for whatever it was you had?" "Yes," I replied tersely, "cancer." I now realise he'd been too wrapped up in his own life to take in what had taken place in mine, and that there was nothing I could do about that. I've expected people to react in a certain way, as if there's only one acceptable way to react when someone's had a life-threatening disease. I know now that it won't always happen the way I want it to, and through talking about that at Life Force I've been able to realise that everybody's different and responds to these things in their own way.

As my first six-monthly check-up approached, I could talk at Life Force meetings about my fears, or my lack of fear at times, or even about the fact that yes, I actually gained a sneaky bit of pleasure from any attention I gained from having had cancer. This only added to my confused feelings, but through verbalising it I could see it for what it was and separate what was helpful and what was not. Apparently, studies have shown it's not an unusual reaction, and I don't need to compound it by feeling guilty about it. But talking about it helps me to let go of it.

I was also able to confront powerful feelings that I had to accomplish everything I'd ever wanted to do — right now. I wanted to be an award-winning novelist, I wanted to be super-fit and I didn't want to spend time with people I no longer cared for or waste time on doing mundane things like working at jobs I didn't enjoy. What if life all ended tomorrow?

Well, just because I've had cancer, that doesn't change the fact that I only have so many hours in the day, I'm not an elite athlete, I have awkward friendships to maintain, and I need to pay my bills.

True, I do spend more time doing things I really want to do and yes, there are times when *carpe diem* or 'seize the day' is the only right response. I'm not about to climb Mount Everest, because that's not my style. But I actually am writing a novel (free from expectation of what will become of it). I do a lot of exercise. I eat healthily. I try to avoid people I dislike. And I try not to do work that I really, really hate.

Yet there are also many times when, for me at least, the only right response is to go to work even when it seems tedious, perform mundane activities like keeping a tidy home, put work into friendships through all their ups and downs and, most importantly, there are times when I need to take things easy and not expect too much of myself and if that means lying on the sofa with a DVD and packet of M&Ms, then that's just fine.

Cancer gave me simultaneous urges to be reckless and ultra-careful, and, through going to Life Force, I've been able to balance those contradictory forces, in the knowledge that yes, my cancer could return one day but that actually it might not. The wonderful thing now is that I'm in extremely capable hands, in the form of the excellent urologist who performed the original surgery, and that every decision I make is informed by the awareness of what might have been if I hadn't decided to deal with a minor embarrassment on August 26, 2005.

Since that day, I've had four check-ups. Naturally, each time I've wanted the doctor to tell me, "Oh yes, all clear!" That hasn't been the case. The first time he said, "Ah, I can see a slight thickening of the bladder wall. It could be an early sign of recurrence. Next time we'll do a biopsy." Six months later, the biopsy was all clear. Six months later, the thickening was still there. Six months later he did another biopsy — again all-clear.

One day, perhaps, there'll be no more thickening. I don't know. But throughout all this, and the accompanying fears it brings up, I've lived my life, gone to the gym, ridden my bike, studied, worked, made progress on my book, gone for dinner, to the movies, on holiday, bought clothes, acquired Marcus and Will (two boisterous kittens), paid my home loan each fortnight and visited my family in the UK. I wouldn't have been able to do any of that without Life Force.

Whenever I have a check-up, I now take the following day off work — and I spend it at the beach, having a massage, going to the gym, doing whatever feels right for me at the time. There's more than one way to seize the day, and I've discovered that kicking back is a great way to do it.

Have I asked anyone out on a date? Yes, I have — and I've been rejected! (More gratifyingly, I've also been asked out.) Will I travel to South America on my own? Possibly. Will I jump out of a plane? I doubt it — heights aren't really my thing. And why would I need to? My life is grand as it is.

Nurturing the Whole

Pat Woolford

I cannot separate my cancer journey with that of Life Force. The two go together and Life Force softened the experience in numerous ways. I was so very fortunate to have a hospital social worker march into the room on my first chemotherapy session and thrust forms and pamphlets into my hand, amongst which was one for the Life Force cancer support group meetings. She did not have more than a few minutes to stop and talk but she had enough time to tell me that the groups were very worthwhile and that she recommended them. How grateful I am to her, especially as I have since found out that it is not at all routine for new patients to be informed of the existence of Life Force, let alone to have it recommended.

It was late February 2002 when I returned one Sunday afternoon from a two-week holiday in New Zealand. I worked part-time, three days a week, as a community mental health nurse in an inner city team. I had reduced my working hours several years before after some back injuries. The reduced hours had restored my health and I was enjoying life to the full. I had enough money to live comfortably and to take occasional trips, especially if I could take advantage of staying with friends, which is what I did in Auckland on this trip. I hired a car and travelled north and also went for many long walks along waterfronts, beaches and through the city gardens and markets. I was a little tired but that was nothing out of the ordinary.

At 51 years old I considered myself fairly fit under the circumstances. I had been diagnosed with thyroid disease at the age of 45 which had taken a toll on my health in some respects. The main problem had been that the disease had caused considerable weight gain. This weight gain had been exacerbated by the minimal activity levels forced on me after lower back injuries caused by work-related falls. Nevertheless, I was enjoying life very much, living in a unit on the harbour where I had lived for over 25 years, with an adult son living away from home, catching up with friends regularly, seeing movies often, reading and generally participating in inner city Sydney living.

The day after I returned from New Zealand, a Monday, I got in the shower getting ready to go to work and felt large lumps on both sides of my neck. I was bemused. They had not been there the night before. I did not begin to guess what it might mean. I went to work and ignored it for the day. I ignored it for two days and then on the Wednesday decided to act. My general practitioner happened to be away for that week, a highly unusual occurrence. For some unknown reason I ended up in a suburb I never normally go to and walked in off the street into a medical centre. To my eternal good fortune I was taken seriously, sent immediately for x-rays and an ultrasound and within days had been diagnosed with non-Hodgkin's lymphoma. I have heard so many tales of people with lymphoma waiting months and even years to get a proper diagnosis that I cannot believe I was so fortunate to have been taken seriously so quickly. I was referred to a surgeon, had a biopsy, tests and the usual round of pre-treatment rigmarole which in total took seven weeks before I was placed on CHOP chemotherapy (Cyclophosphamide/Vincristine/Adriamycin/Prednisone). Again, I was very fortunate to have such a dedicated surgeon that he even saw me in his private rooms on Good Friday.

That whole period is not only a blur now it was a blur at the time. I know I took up the offer of the Life Force support group straight away and went to the Annandale meeting which was the nearest one to where I live. I have always been the sort of person who liked the group experience and was comfortable to go to a group even if I was new to it. I realise that does not apply to everybody — some groups work and some don't and some work for some people and not others. I went with a completely open mind with no expectations or concerns, just willing to give it a go. The meeting was held in a hall which was in itself fairly ordinary but the two facilitators had made it a welcoming place with candles, soft lighting, a calm, quiet atmosphere with introductions and a respectful ambience. I felt immediately comfortable and accepted. There was no pressure to say anything. One could say as little or as much as one wanted. I don't recall anything I said during this period; rather I recall how much I looked forward to going each week to have that time out from the reality of the cancer diagnosis, the hospital and chemotherapy experience.

Healthwise, I was deteriorating rapidly. Chemotherapy made me sicker each cycle. I was on a regime of three weekly cycles for six cycles in total. I tried desperately to keep my work going but by June had given up all together. Sick leave, annual leave and long service leave kept me going for a few months and then I was on to the Centrelink merry-go-round. I lost all my savings, which had been considerable. My finances became a total mess as I had to renegotiate everything and apply for different rates and exemptions at a time when I was too sick to really deal with so much paperwork. The worst part was that I lived on the top floor of a three floor apartment building and as chemotherapy wore on it became harder and harder to walk and getting up those stairs became like climbing Mount Everest! No matter how hard it was, I would not miss those Thursday night meetings for the support group. They were the one bright light in a week of otherwise tortuous effort of just trying to exist.

One of the worst parts of chemotherapy was my hair falling out but being with a group of other people, some of whom were going through the same experience, made such a difference. Not everybody was going through chemotherapy. Not everybody was currently diagnosed with cancer. Some people were in remission. Occasionally carers were invited to the group if it was a first meeting for a cancer patient. But there was always a feeling that people understood what I was going through even if they weren't in the same place at that time. I would not necessarily be feeling bad about my situation every week. The group was not a sad group with a lot of bad things being talked about. Not at all! Topics could range from the everyday to the uplifting to the depths of feeling. There was often humour and laughter too. Whatever happened I always came away feeling good and feeling glad to have seen the people who were there. Often there would be slightly different people each week. Although they were structured into ten week terms, because of the nature of the group some people were not always well enough to attend each week or others might go away and come back at a later date. It was a living group that changed and grew not just from week to week but from term to term. The two constants were the facilitators, Jane and Caro, and how nice it was to walk in each week and find them calmly sitting there, with the candle lit, waiting for us.

I finished chemotherapy in August 2002. My hair started to grow back even before the last of it had fallen out. In spite of predictions, to my disappointment it did not grow back darker or curly! I put on even more weight as with the metallic taste in my mouth as a side effect of chemotherapy I could not tolerate most foods except dairy foods and I ate mostly cheese, milk, ice cream and chocolate. Disastrous! Worse was to come, as instead of recovering from chemotherapy, as I saw some others do, I was unable to get back any energy. I remained on sick leave from work and on sickness benefits. I kept on going to the groups through into 2003 and really missed it during the break for Christmas and New Year. In June 2003 I was diagnosed with lupus (systemic lupus erythematosis). By that time I was barely able to put one foot in front of the other. I think that may have been when I stopped going to the group as I was physically unable to go anywhere.

I went to a number of the Life Force retreats held at Rootreat near Mudgee in the Central West of New South Wales, three and a half hours drive from Sydney. Held from Friday night to Sunday afternoon in an old stone cottage in a beautiful valley surrounded by trees, birds, gardens with absolute peace and quiet, it was truly a retreat from the cares and worries of having to deal with the fallout of having cancer. The maximum number of people at the retreat was eight, so it was an intimate group and many faces were new to me as not all were from the Annandale group or indeed from the other groups, some came from outside Life Force.

The peace, calm and order of the groups were always transferred to the retreat and the formal activities were balanced with free time in an unhurried way, with yoga, meditation, massages, sand play, vision quest, poetry reading and — on one very special occasion — singing around the piano while one participant played, are some of the memories I have. Wonderful meals prepared by the hosts of Rootreat were superbly healthy as well as delicious which made me feel I wanted to go back home and hold on to that feeling of nurturing both body and soul as long as possible in an optimum way. Of course, the reality of life back home and back in the city was never that ideal but the memories are always precious to me of those retreats. They differ from a holiday. They differ from other indulgences one might give oneself from time to time. It was the holistic nature of the retreat as well as the respectful aura of the weekend (respect for oneself and for the other participants) that made it so different and so special.

Although I was not new to the idea of the group experience, this group was special and different because there was no confrontation. There was no right or wrong. It was a safe place for anybody to say what they felt. It was okay to feel what you were feeling and to say it. The only rules were not to interrupt, speak only for oneself and not to put anybody down. There was order to proceedings. Everybody had a turn to say something. It was not a free-for-all. That meant there was no domination by more articulate people. More importantly, if one felt like not talking at all one night that was alright too. The respect for people's feelings was paramount and that was very powerful. It created in me a sense of calm and order when my life was in chaos and disintegration. Not only for the two hours of the group meeting did I know I could gain that sense of control but I knew that I could look forward to that again week after week, for as long as I wanted to continue. I also knew that I was with people who understood my experience in a way that friends or family couldn't, however much they cared about what was happening to me. That was also very important.

Attending the Annandale group gave me an opportunity to evaluate my attitude to death, not just other people's dying but the possibility of my own early mortality. There have been many positive outcomes for me of this process including writing out my life story for my son, which would never have occurred to me to do before this experience. I place a greater value on being in the present and valuing peace and harmony than I did before. That is partly because I am no longer able to work and was forced to retire early because of my illness but I also feel my experience with Life Force, through the Annandale group meetings and the retreats, has helped to give me the tools to do this. My attitude to death and dying has changed as a result of being exposed to the possibility, and in many cases the reality, that death can be achieved with peace, care, respect and love, if only the right attitude is there in the people one is surrounded by.

I still maintain contact with Life Force even though I no longer attend the group meetings. There are many occasions when I see people from the group and the facilitators and I feel I still have a connection with Life Force and that I always will. The hospital experience is one of being a number and the file gets shut once treatment is finished and one feels left out in the cold in so many ways. I am very grateful to still be in remission and I have no complaints about the doctors and nurses I saw. However, regardless of how nice they may be, they can never leave you feeling nurtured in the way I felt through my contact with Life Force, both with the other members of the group (and at the retreats) and with the facilitators. I was indeed fortunate to have met that social worker that frightening day I first started chemotherapy. How one small contact can lead to so much still amazes me.

Why Me?

Shirley Cottle

Television actress Belinda Emmett's sad death from breast cancer reminded me again of all the wonderful women who have fought so bravely against this terrible disease. I do not count myself among them because I was filled with terror, hatred and anger after being diagnosed. I didn't feel at all brave.

I had rolled over in bed one night and felt a lump on the side of my breast. "Oh, a gland, I thought," and didn't really think about it anymore. However, I did mention it to my daughter, Charlotte, who said, "You'd better have that checked out." A few days later I happened to be passing a hospital and saw the NSW Breast Screening sign outside. So on the spur of the moment, I went in and had a mammogram, then went on holiday to Turkey.

What I didn't know until I returned was that my lump was suspicious and an appointment had been made for me for a repeat mammogram. After that it was all out of my hands. I had breast cancer. I saw surgeons, oncologists and radiation specialists and one week later had a lumpectomy to be followed by radiation and chemotherapy.

I was unprepared for my life to skid out of control. I was unprepared for my anger and depression. I'm ashamed to say I hated healthy people. I wanted to know, "Why me?" I spent my days flat on my back looking at the ceiling or the palm trees against the blue sky in the park, feeling so ill after the chemo and radiation that I could barely move. I wouldn't have moved at all, except for the necessity of crossing Sydney for treatment.

About a year before my diagnosis, my daughter had moved

out of our flat to be with her fiancé and they moved to the country for work. Taking her place came my friend, Jane Gillespie, newly arrived from Canberra. When I first met Jane she was desperately struggling to learn how to make a different life for herself after treatment for her breast cancer. Jane was like a gift from God at that time. My daughter was still on her way to Sydney, so Jane drove me to hospital for surgery and held my hand as I was wheeled down to the operating theatre. I was touched that she bought me a magazine to read after the operation. I was very frightened. Was I going to come out of this alive?

When I was well enough, Jane drove me to Life Force meetings with Jilly and Caro and other cancer patients. I was not alone any more. I met some wonderful brave people who wanted so desperately to live and fought so hard to do so. Val, with the flaming red hair, who would not give up but, finally, was taken by this terrible disease; Noelle, a lovely young woman, honoured and loved by the homeless at the Wayside Chapel; Angie, who went into Sacred Heart Hospice to die but couldn't leave her young son alone, so she postponed dying; Chris who came to a retreat using an oxygen tank; and Margaret, who loved to laugh and share a whisky on the veranda at Kandos, where Life Force retreats are held.

The retreats are exceptional gatherings. I expected to be depressed and instead was surrounded with laughter and love. After being warmly welcomed by hosts John and Jolieske, I will always remember sitting down in the lovely country kitchen to huge breakfasts prepared by John, who always had something to say as he cooked, and later enjoying a delicious dinner with wine. Those meals were really special times together and during the day there was the opportunity to enjoy yoga, massages, and other activities and, for me, painting on the veranda and later in the evening, looking at the endless starlit sky with the others.

All cancer patients live with the Sword of Damocles over our heads. Will the cancer return? I don't know. The thought is ever there in the background and I do try and check regularly. Friends have been told by their doctors to go away and not think about it (not my surgeon and oncologist by the way, who tell me to check regularly), but can we ever do that? Whenever something happens to my body, and friends who have suffered cancer tell me they feel the same way, immediately we fearfully consult our doctors. Unfortunately we will never be completely free.

I'm not sure how I could have managed to get through those months of treatment, except for the friendship and support I received from weekly Life Force meetings and weekends at the wonderful retreats.

A Year Out of My Life

Deidre Pinder

When I first got out of hospital after my double mastectomy for breast cancer the community nurse advised me to allow a year of my life to get through the whole treatment process. This story is therefore about that year out of my life. It is about my cancer journey, the experience and emotions involved. Interspersed throughout this story are tips of what I've learnt and that helped me get through.

It began like this: One Thursday morning in late August 2009 whilst showering I lifted up my right arm to wash my breast and found a lump on top. A cold chill ran down my back as this felt like a serious lump.

I made a GP appointment. As I waited I found it hard to believe that it is anything. Only other people get cancer and cancer simply didn't run on my mother's side of the family. Nope I was low risk. I wouldn't have cancer. It would be nothing, probably a cyst.

My GP examined my breast and agreed that indeed there was a lump. She referred me for an ultrasound. I took the referral, guessing it was time I had a breast ultrasound as I haven't had one for several years and have had problems with micro-calcifications and cysts in the past.

After my investigations, I'm given an envelope with my results and advised to see my GP. I take it home. In spite of a tag saying, "Must be opened by GP only", I opened it up and read the report. It talked of extensive micro-calcification and advised the results are strongly indicative of malignancy for both breasts. It recommended a specialist referral. I gasped in horror. I knew what 'malignancy' meant, it was a fancy word for cancer. I examined the films but they meant nothing. I kept re-reading report. I googled the terms in the report.

I told my partner what it said and that it doesn't look good. The clock ticks by, three hours from finding out, four hours, five hours since finding out.

Questions spun around my head. Would I need a mastectomy? Would it be a double mastectomy? It looked fairly widespread. There wouldn't be much breast left by the looks of things. A mastectomy sounded like an awfully painful process to go through. Will it mean chemo, which involved hideous illness and violent vomiting? How would I work? I had absolutely no other means of support other than what I earn through my labour. I guessed I would have to just take a bucket to work.

When I was out at the shops I bumped into the local breast screen van. At home I found a pink breast cancer shopping bag. And there was a bottle of mineral water in the fridge with a pink lid on it. It seemed very in my face all of a sudden.

I faxed off the report to my GP who refered me for a fine needle biopsy.

On Thursday 10 September 2009 my GP called me at work. "I'd like you to come and see me right away. It's not good news."

That was also the day my manager found out as I felt I had to explain why I needed to leave the office immediately, in tears. Thankfully my workplace was very supportive, never acting as if my cancer was an inconvenience or difficulty, instead reassuring me that I could have whatever time off I needed and they would give their full support.

Afterwards I sat at home and wondered that if the lump had not come up how long it would have taken for it to have killed me. Would it have been two years? How would I have known? Would I have suddenly collapsed one day to find I was riddled with it? Was I already riddled with it? Every ache seemed ominous.

I had further biopsies and saw the surgeon who recommended a double mastectomy followed by chemotherapy. Radiotherapy would depend on whether there was lymph node involvement. A surgery date was set. As I felt the surgery recommended was in keeping with what I'd expected I didn't feel a need to seek a second opinion.

Tip: Do your medical research.

Tip: Take someone with you to at least key appointments.

Tip: Don't be afraid to seek a second opinion if you aren't happy with the treatment options recommended or you're on the borderline of two treatment options.

I had a lot of immediate decisions to make and things to organise as I was working part-time whilst studying occupational therapy at university. With work I didn't have much sick leave accrued and with the huge gaps in Australia's welfare net I was not eligible for any payment from Centrelink. Thus continuing to work through treatment was my first priority. Also in my mind people with cancer did not work so if I went to work then it meant that I did not have cancer — well at least for the time I was at work.

I could have withdrawn from my studies, however I had completed so much of the term that I decided to continue on. This meant putting in for special consideration. At the same time I studied while in hospital waiting rooms, when recovering from surgery and even on the bus to and from the hospital and work. I did miss lectures as tests clashed with work and lectures which meant swapping work days when needed, leading to more missed lectures. However, extra study paid off with passes in all subjects.

It can takes weeks to know the type, grade and extent of the cancer, so making decisions can be difficult. When and how does one tell friends, relatives and colleagues? Future treatment can only be guessed at until the full pathology report is available a week after surgery. My supervisor at work wanted to let staff in my section know but I wanted to wait until I had the full information. We did agree that it would be best that I not be present when he told the other staff.

With my friends I made decisions on an individual basis about whether to tell them face to face, via email or via telephone. After the initial notification I decided to provide email updates at regular intervals. One friend upon receiving my news via email called me leaving a message saying, "Please ring me," rather than replying via email. Another friend who has various health problems pulled out all stops to visit me in hospital.

At the same time a couple of friendships ended. However friends who were difficult to catch up with prior to my diagnosis now catch up with me regularly. My cancer has brought home that keeping up with friends is important as they may not be around one day.

Tip: Communicate with family, friends and workmates early about your needs and how best they can support you. Consider sending group email updates as people like to hear how you are going and feel less awkward if they know what you want from them. Consider sending the Breast Cancer Network Australia brochure on how to talk to your friend or colleague about their breast cancer.

One thing I did find hard was hearing stories of how the 'community' pulled together to support the person, always providing transport, house cleaning and meals. Even though we had some good friends, they had moved away several years before so weren't easily available to help out. I had no close family on my side. Our friendly neighbours on each side had sold up to be replaced by people who weren't interested. Thankfully we had a great set of shopkeepers who cared and I met some great people through my journey.

Suddenly it was Thursday 15 October — double mastectomy day. I shuffled off to hospital with my partner and his mother and sister fearing that I may either not wake up at all or wake up from the general anesthetic as a vegetable or totally paralysed. Thankfully once I was in the operating room things moved too quickly for me to worry. I was soon waking up but I made sure that no one was looking when I lifted the sheet to check that "they had gone".

By this stage I'd been contacted by a breast care nurse. I assumed she was there only to change dressings post surgery. However, I soon found out that she was a counselor and educator, and I wished I'd contacted her earlier. Like a guardian angel she was there every step of the way ordering me breast care kits, visiting me in hospital, showing me what prosthetic breasts looked like and letting me know what supports were available including the Life Force Cancer Foundation support and Encore breast exercise groups.

Tip: Take advantage of any support available including care nurses, counsellors and support groups. Even if you need to try a few support groups to find one that's right for you, the effort is worth it. Getting support for yourself will also make it easier for those who care and support you.

After four days and with three drains I was discharged home from hospital. A community nurse was sent to manage my drains. I had an appointment with the surgeon the following Thursday.

I went shopping as many of my old clothes simply did not suit or fit. To my surprise there was virtually no information on what I called 'post-mastectomy dressing'. Sure there were prosthesis and reconstruction but what about those who don't always want to wear prosthesis or when it's too soon after surgery?

I also avoided looking at my chest. Every time I showered I would fog up the bathroom so I couldn't see myself in the mirror naked. But over several days I gradually worked up my courage to look at my chest initially starting off with looking down at it and then through a less foggy mirror. So it didn't come as quite of a shock. Seeing pictures of mastectomy scars prior to surgery also helped.

A week post surgery I met with the surgeon, who advised me that there had been DCIS in the left breast, invasive ductal carcinoma in my right with extensive lymph node involvement. Thus I would need radiotherapy as well as chemotherapy. He referred me to the medical oncologist to plan chemotherapy, and for blood tests, a full body bone and CT scan.

I asked how long the cancer had been there and he replied one to two years. The answer came as a shock as just over two years before I'd been for a PAP smear with a different GP who had failed to do a breast check or take a breast history. The examination and history would have created enough concern to have referred me for tests which would have picked up the cancer at pre-cancer DCIS stage in both breasts meaning only surgery and a near 100 per cent survival rate.

I returned to work a couple of weeks after surgery with one drain still *in situ*. The community nurse suggested I get a bum-bag which did the trick.

The next step was the oncologist to discuss chemotherapy. I sat waiting, hoping that the oncologist didn't decide that I was a hopeless case and deemed not suitable for treatment. I also wondered how I could make a good impression on this person who was going to be responsible for me hopefully having a very long life. This was someone I definitely wanted on my side. I had the results of my bone and CT scans with me but was afraid to open them up in case it said bad things such as, "patient is riddled with cancer and thus a hopeless case". Ironically it was Melbourne Cup day so I wondered if I would be a good horse to make a bet on.

Tip: Take someone with you to at least key appointments.

The oncologist told then me my scans were clear. It was the first bit of good news I'd had for a while. In spite of my fear that treatment may not be deemed necessary due to a possible anxiety disorder I advised the oncologist of my full medical history.

The oncologist said I would need to have chemotherapy. The treatment would be AC (Adriamycin and Cyclophosphamide) every three weeks for four cycles then twelve weekly sessions of Taxol, Herceptin or Tykerb as my tumor was HER2 positive. The oncologist advised me to work Mondays to Wednesdays, have chemo on the Thursday and rest on the Friday. A chemo start date was set for the day after my last university exam.

Tip: If you have to work accessing flexible hours and part-time working arrangements will really help you get through.

On the first day of chemo my partner and I presented nervously at the hospital. After this first session I needed to have a blood test at least 90 minutes prior to seeing the doctor who then decides whether I'm fit to have chemo or not. But on this first day with bloods already taken by the surgeon I get straight into it. I've had to get prescriptions made up for Emend, Dexamethasone and Maxolon which all prevent nausea and vomiting.

A nurse directed me to take the Emend for the nausea then explained the side effects, what to watch out for, when to contact them and other instructions.

They started to infuse the medicine and I felt sick. Then I was told it was just the pre-med and I realised I was actually feeling hungry.

Around three hours later it was all done and we're ready to go.

We went out for lunch, did a little shopping and then went home. I sat around for the rest of the day waiting for a reaction. I did develop a headache and called the hospital to ask if I could take a Panadol. But overall I was pleased that the horrid vomiting I'd associated with chemotherapy had not occurred.

The following Monday, which was also the day that I stopped the main anti-nausea medications, I went back to work. I felt both nauseous and fatigued, and had to keep taking Maxolon tablets to keep the nausea at bay. I wondered if I was actually meant to do this but was saved by someone offering to buy coffees. Even though I was trying to avoid non-essential drugs such as caffeine I decided to accept the coffee and it worked.

I made it through the other three chemotherapy sessions. Even though I didn't get violently ill or vomit I did find it a struggle for up to two weeks after each treatment. I felt fatigued, nauseous and mentally flat. Before each treatment I would lay out my clothes for work for the following week to save me the effort on work mornings. Sometimes I needed to take a sick day or swap a working day. Once on the weekly Taxol treatment it was less taxing, which made working easier.

Tip: Don't think in absolutes, for example, about whether you need to either totally work or totally not work through treatment. You can always have time off or work part-time for parts of treatment whilst returning to part-time or full-time work for other parts.

My hair did fall out just after the second treatment. Knowing this would happen I had cut my hair short in preparation and had brought a couple of wigs online. But it was still a shock.

Tip: Don't be tempted to buy wigs online, do go into wig places and actually try the wig on. Then you know if the wig will suit you. They can also trim it up for you. It's also an opportunity to try something daring such as a completely different colour, as the staff can ensure the right colour match.

Up until chemotherapy I hadn't really met any others undergoing cancer treatment. I'd never spent much time in hospital waiting rooms either. However once I'd started treatment I quickly met other patients who wanted to chat and swap stories. One time while waiting to see the oncologist a conversation broke out between the women in the seats near me. One of these women would end up becoming a good friend. As it was obviously an open group I joined in. We were so busy swapping stories that we were disappointed when the oncologists started calling us in. During my consultation I could hear the rest of the group laughing through the closed door and knowing I was part of that group gave me a warm feeling.

Tip: Use coming in contact with other patients as an opportunity to connect. No one else except another cancer patient truly knows what you are going through and you may meet some amazing people.

During chemotherapy I began to attend support groups and cancer information sessions including sessions about finances, legalities and employment issues. I was shocked to hear how difficult it was to access superannuation even when considered terminally ill. A person needs to be within one year of death to gain access. Prior to the cancer I had felt it was a good thing to contribute additional payments to my superannuation but I now don't as I feel the money is better off in my bank account where I can access it.

After chemotherapy I had six weeks of daily radiotherapy. In spite of the hassle of treatment prior to work on some days the time flew by and suddenly it was over. Then came the wondering. Will it come back? When will it come back? Where? How will I know that it's come back? It seemed to crawl around my breast for an awfully long period of time before it became apparent! Thus how will I know early if it does come back? I worry that cells could be gathering in a part of my body forming into a tumor even as I type now.

I asked the oncologist what symptoms I needed to look out for and he said pain, nausea, bloating, breathlessness, loss of appetite and weight loss. So, most mornings I check to see if I have any of these symptoms.

It's now the end of this 'year of my life' and I'm slowly getting on with things and making the most of every day. I don't think too far into the future but live for the present. I have gone back to my studies and even got some temporary work in the disability field. I'm involved in some volunteer work for a community organisation and started up a Facebook cancer social group. I see my friends regularly and have taken up photography.

And now I will leave you with some final tips for getting through the experience:

- Contact relevant cancer organisation helplines.
- Attend any cancer related educational courses.
- Read information contained on cancer websites. This will help you in a whole lot of areas including access to superannuation/income protection/disability payouts, Centrelink entitlements, managing work, treatment options as well as dealing with the psychosocial impacts such as managing relationships and sexuality.
- Ensure you schedule regular pleasurable activities into your life. It's easy to let these activities go when you are caught up in doctor and treatment visits.
- Be kind to yourself.

Recommended Reading

Beck, Martha, *Finding Your Own North Star*, 2001. Piatkus Books

Cameron, Julia, *The Artist's Way*, 1999. Self published by Julia Cameron and Mark Bryan

Chapman, Gary, *The Five Love Languages*, 2000. Strand Publishing

His Holiness the Dalai Lama and Cutler MD, Howard C, *The Art of Happiness—A Handbook For Living*, 2000. Hodder

Ferruci, Piero, *What We May Be*, 1982. Aquarian/Thorsons

Harpham, Wendy Schlessel, *After Cancer*, 1995. William Morrow and Company

Holland, Jimmie C, Lewis, Sheldon, *The Human Side of Cancer*, 2000. HarperCollins

National Coalition for Cancer Survivorship; *A Cancer Survivor's Almanac;* edited by Barbara Hoffman, 1996

Kuhl, David, *What Dying People Want*, 2002. Perseus Books Group

Kessler, David: *The Rights of the Dying*, 1997. HarperCollins

Leimbach, Claire; McShane, Trypheyna; Virago, Zenith, *The Intimacy of Death and Dying*, 2009. Allen and Unwin

Lerner, Harriet, *The Dance of Anger*, 1985, 1997. HarperCollins

Longaker, Christine, *Facing Death and Finding Hope*, 1998. Crown Publishing Group

Myss, Caroline, *Anatomy of the Spirit — The Seven Stages of Power and Healing*, 1996. Bantam Books

Somers, Suzanne, *Ageless*, 2006. Three Rivers Press

Wilbur, Ken, *Grace and Grit*, 2000. Shambala Publications

Wolfelt, Alan D, *Understanding Your Grief*, 2003. Companion Press

The Person Behind
the Meditations — Caro Jonas

Meldi Arkinstall

Caro Jonas' life philosophy is one which values harmony and balance, with a deep spiritual base and connection to nature.

Her philosophy of life has been influenced by two people: Joseph Campbell and Dr Phillip Groves. Ideas generated by reading work by Campbell and through attending discussion groups led by Dr Philip Groves laid a foundation upon which Caro began to write her own meditations.

Campbell taught mythology at Sarah Lawrence College in New York for 38 years and was one of the great thinkers of his time. When journalist Bill Moyers met him, he decided to write a book on Campbell called *The Power of Myth*. This book profoundly influenced many people, including filmmaker George Lucas, who paid homage to the book in his movie series *Star Wars*.

The idea of the pollen path is discussed by Campbell in depth in *The Power of Myth*. He believed the journey was more important than the destination and referred to the Navaho Indians to whom pollen was the life source. The pollen path was the path to the centre.

Thus the 'Pollen Path' or Tadidiin bee Kek'ehashchiin, is a metaphor for 'travelling'; for moving along one's life trail. A poem by the Navaho Indians describes the importance of pollen and how it is everywhere:

Oh, beauty before me,
beauty behind me,
beauty to the right of me,
beauty to the left of me,
beauty below me,
I am on the pollen path.

Caro sees her life as a pollen path, a path that started at the Battle of Britain. It was there her parents met and fell in love. Her English mother was a plotter of enemy aircraft; her New Zealand father was a tail gunner on a Lancaster bomber.

Having survived the war, her parents moved to New Zealand and her two younger sisters, Maggy and Andy were born there.

New Zealand was a safe and idyllic place to grow up. But they were about to be hit with a bombshell.

"We had a comfortable middle-class existence. Then, when I was nineteen, my mother killed herself by jumping off the Auckland Bridge", she said.

Attempting to deal with the painful emotional ravages of her mother's suicide, she travelled to England.

In London she gained employment as a waitress at Ronnie Scott's famous jazz club where she rubbed shoulders with some of the great entertainers of the day, including Janis Joplin, Jimi Hendricks, The Beatles, Osibisa, Lou Rawls, Miles Davis, Thelonius Monk, Dizzy Gillespie, Stan Getz and Sonny Rollins. The comedian Spike Milligan became a good friend, and she socialised with Peter Sellers and jazz great Blossom Dearie.

The club was the place to be in London. Celebrities, royalty and gangsters all converged on it to see, be seen and to hear great music. She spent six years immersed in its culture.

"The Cray twins, the notorious London gangsters, came in one night — such evil, with such sweet faces. Also Frank Sinatra's entourage came in, about ten of them, in very expensive suits. They ordered everything in sight, consumed it all and signed a tab for it. We knew that they would never pay; and … they didn't."

Caro recall one particularly memorable night when Peter Sellers came in.

"He was accompanied by Princess Margaret, with whom he was allegedly having an affair at the time," Caro recalled.

"They were sitting at their table trying to be anonymous when Ronnie Scott, the owner, a great jazz player in his own right and a famous wit, while he was onstage said in a rhyme:

Whoever you are, wherever you may be,
Please take your hand off the princess's knee.

"The place erupted with laughter. What a moment."

This exciting life helped soften the traumatic memories of what happened to her mother, "for a little while at least".

The creative world of jazz opened her mind and she began reading widely: Jung, Gurdjieff, and Herman Hess, Victor Frankl, Maurice Nicholl, John Bennett, Rumi, Ouspensky, Swedenborg and the like.

Turning to Buddhist meditation she discovered an ability to focus the mind, to concentrate on the breath, and she found a peace that she had never found before. Step by step she was healing.

Moving to Sydney in 1971 to join her family, Caro met her husband Stephen Leeder in 1976 and they've been together ever since.

"Throughout all he has been my love and greatest support."

Through meeting Stephen she started attending lectures by Dr Philip Groves in Sydney.

Dr Groves held PhDs in biochemistry, psychology and divinity, was a qualified and practising naturopath and psychotherapist, and had extensive knowledge of Egyptology, comparative religion and natural sciences.

Dr Groves' teachings had a profound impact on Caro.

The foundation of his teaching, which spanned more than 40 years before he died in 1999, was to encourage a sense of the abundance of life, creative expression and the development of a deeper knowledge and understanding of the world in which we live.

Topics explored included esoteric Christianity, Sufism, and the works of Gurdjieff and Emanuel Swedenborg, as well as science, history, botany and psychology.

"It was a closed group. I had to wait six months before I could attend. He interviewed me and decided I was ready," Caro said.

"If you want something, if you search it out, you will find it. That's the approach Dr Groves took: his lectures were open to people who were truly searching."

In his book, *The Garden of the Mind,* Groves explores the connection between the divine and nature, particularly gardens.

"The ancients realised that order and harmony are not accidental, self-generated principles, but depict the way in which Divine intelligence or wisdom generates and sustains creation … so as to represent to themselves an image of creative intelligence, the ancients selected the symbol of the garden."

Caro uses gardens and other outdoor settings as the basis of a number of her meditations. The visualisations contained in these meditations are powerful and symbolic, and are inspired by Groves' teachings.

Describing the "almost universal urge to construct gardens", Groves explains that for many people a beautiful garden suggests another-worldly state.

Xenophon and other Greeks who visited Persia and Assyria saw the gardens there and described them as *paradeisoi.*

Egyptians were aware of the spiritual significance of gardens and travelled to distant lands to collect aromatic plants. The

Romans saw the benefits of Grecian gardens and developed their own villas and elaborate gardens. Some noble families took their names from the plants they proudly cultivated. The Valerii from *Valerians* and the Lactuciui from *Lactuca*, the lettuce.

Groves explained the benefits of visualising a garden within oneself: we can keep watch on the truths we plant in the soil of the spirit and observe how they grow, flower and bear fruit from our repeated contemplations ... a well-watered garden is an active, awakened mind that forever increases in wisdom, love, understanding, purity of motive and constancy of will.

Caro's artistic nature also led her to study art for seven years at East Sydney Tech (now the National Art School). She studied painting, photography, etching, drawing, sculpture, printmaking, art theory, colour and design.

One of her paintings, a portrait of Dr Phillip Groves, was chosen to hang for the Blake Prize for Religious Art in 1994.

The next step in the pollen path involved a long time friend calling Caro for help. Jilly Pascoe had been friends with Caro for years and knew of her lifelong interest in meditation. Jilly had cancer and thought meditating would help with managing the plethora of emotions she was experiencing.

They began meditating and visualising together, and Jilly found it hugely beneficial.

Jilly felt that after people finished treatment and left the hospital, there was little available to help deal with things emotionally. The duo decided to start support groups to fill the gap. It was 1993 and Life Force had begun; another major step on Caro's pollen path.

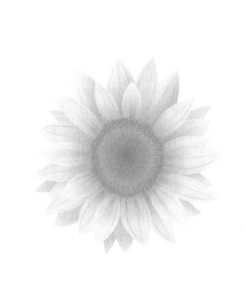